Parkinson's Disease

YOUR QUESTIONS ANSWERED

For Churchill Livingstone

Commissioning Editor: Ellen Green
Project Development and Management: Fiona Conn
Design: Jayne Jones, George Ajayi, Keith Kail
Illustrator: Bruce Hogarth

Parkinson's Disease

YOUR QUESTIONS ANSWERED

Thomas Foltynie
MB BS, MRCP, MPHIL
Clinical Research Registrar,
Cambridge Centre for Brain Repair,
Addenbrooke's Hospital,
Cambridge, UK

Simon Lewis
MB BS
Clinical Research Registrar,
Cambridge Centre for Brain Repair,
Addenbrooke's Hospital,
Cambridge, UK

Roger A. Barker
MB BS, MRCP
MRC Clinician Scientist and Honorary Consultant in Neurology,
Cambridge Centre for Brain Repair,
Addenbrooke's Hospital,
Cambridge, UK

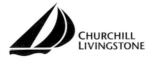
CHURCHILL
LIVINGSTONE

EDINBURGH LONDON NEW YORK PHILADELPHIA ST LOUIS SYDNEY TORONTO 2003

CHURCHILL LIVINGSTONE
An imprint of Elsevier Science Limited

First published 2003

ISBN 0 433 06417 2

British Library Cataloguing in Publication Data
A catalogue record for this book is available from the British Library

Library of Congress Cataloging in Publication Data
A catalog record for this book is available from the Library of Congress

Note
Medical knowledge is constantly changing. As new information becomes
available, changes in treatment, procedures, equipment and the use of
drugs become necessary. The authors and the publishers have taken care
to ensure that the information given in this text is accurate and up to
date. However, readers are strongly advised to confirm that the
information, especially with regard to drug usage, complies with the latest
legislation and standards of practice.

**ELSEVIER
SCIENCE**
your source for books,
journals and multimedia
in the health sciences
www.elsevierhealth.com

The
publisher's
policy is to use
paper manufactured
from sustainable forests

Printed in China by RDC Group Limited

Contents

Preface

Parkinson's disease (PD) is a relatively uncommon disease, but it is common enough that most general practitioners will have to consider the diagnosis or treat patients with it at some point. A practice of multiple partners serving in the region of 10 000 patients is likely to have about 10–20 patients with symptoms of PD at any one time. Some of these patients will be independent and still working, whereas others might be in residential care or nursing homes. As a result, it takes many years for an individual GP to build up a broad experience of treating the different phases of this disorder. In addition, the continued research into PD makes it difficult to keep up with new developments relevant to patient care.

For these reasons, we have composed a series of questions to act as a source of reference for GPs involved in the care of PD patients. The book is not structured like a traditional textbook, but is hopefully arranged in a logical order, addressing issues that might arise both within and outside a patient consultation. Emphasis has been placed on information most relevant to a GP, with brief references to the more minor aspects of neurological diagnosis. We hope, however, to have included sufficient information to enable a GP to happily manage patients when neurological referral is not possible or desirable, as well as provide the necessary background to follow and understand the management of patients in specialist hospital clinics. Brief answers to questions are included in addition to more complete answers. At the end of each chapter a selection of common patient questions and possible answers to them have also been included.

Whilst we hope that the questions and answers in this book are relevant, we are only too aware of the fact that not all questions that could be asked have been addressed. Furthermore, we have had to be didactic in our answers, as books of this nature inevitably require such an approach. However, we have acknowledged where there is insufficient evidence to answer a question or advise on management.

We hope that you find the book helpful, but are always keen to hear if there are areas that we have neglected or misrepresented.

Tom Foltynie
Simon Lewis
Roger Barker

Portrait

How to use this book

The *Your Questions Answered* series aims to meet the information needs of GPs and other primary care professionals who care for patients with chronic conditions. It is designed to help them work with patients and their families, providing effective, evidence-based care and management.

The books are in an accessible question and answer format, with detailed contents lists at the beginning of every chapter and a complete index to help find specific information.

ICONS

Icons are used in the book to identify particular types of information:

 highlights important information

 highlights side-effect information.

PATIENT QUESTIONS

At the end of relevant chapters there are sections of frequently asked patient questions, with easy-to-understand answers aimed at the non-medical reader.

A background knowledge of Parkinson's disease: aetiology, epidemiology and pathology

1

1.1   Who first described Parkinson's disease?

James Parkinson (1817).

Parkinson's disease (PD) takes its name from James Parkinson who in 1817 was the first physician to describe the condition. He coined the term 'paralysis agitans' and described affected individuals as having: 'involuntary tremulous motion, with lessened muscular power, in parts not in action and, even when supported; with a propensity to bend the trunk forwards, and to pass from a walking to a running pace; the senses and intellect being uninjured.'

Subsequently, other doctors especially the famous French neurologist Charcot felt that there were some intellectual impairments associated with the condition and that there were various different types (so called 'formes fruste') of Parkinson's disease.

Many have claimed that the disease was described long before James Parkinson, although who gave the earliest description is somewhat controversial. Galen described shaking occurring in a person while at rest or while carrying out a muscular act, although it was unclear whether he was describing Parkinson's disease. Others have claimed that Leonardo Da Vinci was the first to describe the condition, and evidence from ancient Indian medical texts suggests that the disease may have occurred many years prior to any of these descriptions.

1.2   What is Parkinson's disease?

See Table 1.1.

TABLE 1.1   The defining features of Parkinson's disease

Parkinson's disease is a disorder of unknown cause

With motor symptoms	Pathologically defined by
Tremor at rest (pill-rolling) Slowness of movement Rigidity of the limbs	Presence of Lewy bodies Loss of dopamine in parts of the brain

The current agreed *clinical* definition of Parkinson's disease describes a disorder of unknown cause, characterized by a *tremor that is present at rest*, slowness of movement (*bradykinesia*), stiffness of the muscles (*rigidity*) and impairment of the postural reflexes (leading to falls). These features may be present in varying degrees from one patient to the next and are in some cases accompanied by cognitive abnormalities, which range from subtle frontal lobe deficits to profound dementia.

Several diverse entities, including toxins, pharmacological agents and focal or vascular lesions of the basal ganglia can produce syndromes clinically indistinguishable from PD and these conditions are termed 'secondary parkinsonism'. The range of causes of secondary parkinsonism and the Parkinson-plus syndromes are described in more detail in Chapter 10.

When the brains of Parkinson's disease patients are examined after they have died, selective degeneration of dopaminergic neurons of the substantia nigra pars compacta (SNc) and other brainstem nuclei can be seen. The surviving neurons contain cytoplasmic inclusions (known as Lewy bodies), which stain positively for a protein known as α-synuclein. Follow-up studies that include both clinical information collected during life, and microscopy data at post-mortem show that an initial diagnosis of IPD is inaccurate in 35% of patients, falling to 24% after a mean disease duration of 12 years. Most misdiagnosed patients turn out to have either progressive supranuclear palsy, multiple system atrophy, Alzheimer's disease or vascular parkinsonism (*see Ch. 10* for definitions of these disorders).

Thus the diagnosis of Parkinson's disease can only ever be made *with certainty* at death when the characteristic pathological hallmark of the disease, namely the Lewy body, can be found, especially in the dopamine-rich parts of the brain.

1.3 Are 'Parkinson's disease' and 'idiopathic Parkinson's disease' the same disorder?

Yes.

The definition of Parkinson's disease in the answer to the question above acknowledges the fact that the cause of the disease is unknown, and that it develops for reasons that are not apparent (i.e. idiopathic). Some use the term idiopathic PD to emphasise this point and to distinguish this disorder from parkinsonism caused by a known agent (such as drugs). These latter cases are sometimes known as secondary parkinsonism.

1.4 What is dopamine?

A neurotransmitter in the brain.

Dopamine is a chemical that has a range of functions around the body but has an especially important role as a neurotransmitter in the brain. Dopamine is stored in vesicles in the end of a nerve process and the arrival of an electrical signal down that nerve fibre leads to the vesicles of dopamine being released (*Fig. 1.1*). The dopamine can then either be broken down, or binds to specific sites – the dopamine receptors. The binding of dopamine to these receptors produces an effect in the cell, and if there are

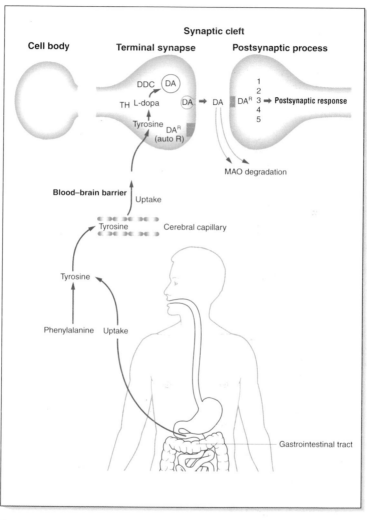

Fig. 1.1 Schematic figure to demonstrate the structure of a dopaminergic synapse, including the synthesis, uptake and metabolism of dopamine. DA, dopamine; TH, tyrosine hydroxylase; DA^R, dopamine receptor; DDC, dopa decarboxylase; MAO, monoamine oxidase; 1–5, five types of dopamine receptor.

no receptors present then dopamine will not have any action. In Parkinson's disease the loss of the dopamine-producing nerves means that whilst the receptors are still present in the brain there is not enough dopamine produced to activate the receptors.

Elsewhere in the body, dopamine has a role in the control of heart rate, blood pressure, and renal function.

1.5 What are the dopamine-rich areas of the brain?

The brainstem – especially the substantia nigra.

There are a number of parts of the brain that are normally rich in dopamine. The majority of nerve cells containing dopamine are found deep within the part of the brainstem known as the midbrain (*see Fig. 1.2*). The dopamine cells in this location send connecting fibres which release dopamine to many different parts of the brain including the outer layer of the brain at the front (frontal cortex), areas involved with emotion and motivation (limbic system) and structures important in movement. These latter structures are called the basal ganglia and receive dopamine projections from the part of the midbrain known as the *substantia nigra*. There are also other areas in the brain that contain dopamine, including the vomiting centre at the bottom of the brain and the hypothalamus–pituitary where it regulates the release of some hormones.

1.6 What are the basal ganglia?

A collection of structures deep within each cerebral hemisphere.

The basal ganglia are a collection of structures found deep within the brain, which are thought to be involved with movement and to a lesser extent thinking. They consist of a number of clear anatomical structures known as the caudate nucleus, putamen, globus pallidus, subthalamic nucleus and substantia nigra. The caudate nucleus and putamen together form the striatum. Abnormalities within these structures can lead to a large number of movement problems including parkinsonism, involuntary abnormal movements such as *chorea* (dance-like movements) and *ballismus* (flailing limb movements). Such involuntary movements are only seen in Parkinson's patients following exposure to drug treatments and are known as dyskinesias (*see Q. 7.11*).

Figure 1.3A shows the connections between the different part of the basal ganglia and Figures 1.3B and C show the appearance of the regions on MRI brain scanning.

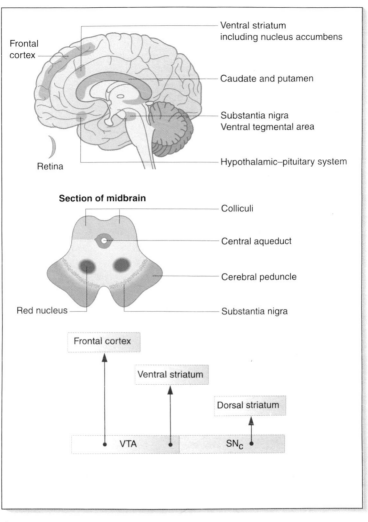

Fig. 1.2 Schematic figure to demonstrate the regions of the brain normally rich in dopamine.

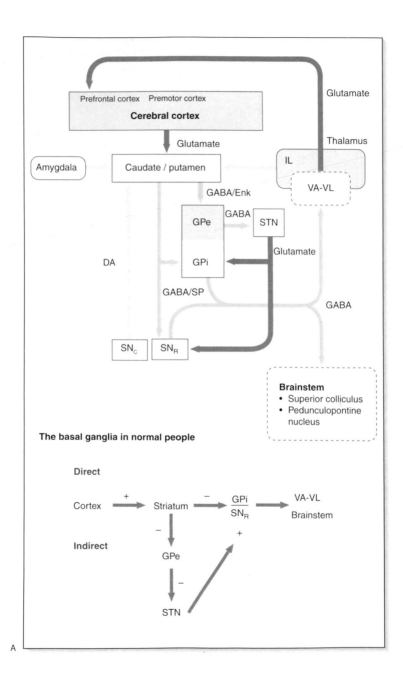

The basal ganglia in normal people

A

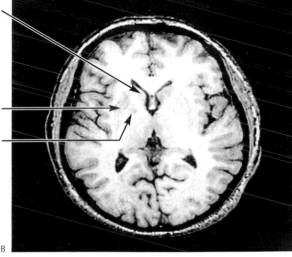

Head of caudate nucleus

Lentiform nucleus
-*Putamen*

-*Globus pallidus*

B

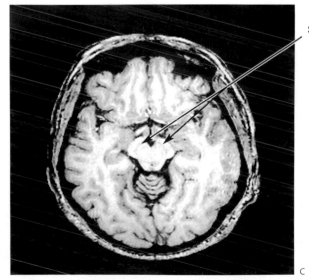

Substantia nigra

C

Fig. 1.3 A. Schematic figure to show the structures and connections that constitute the basal ganglia. **B** and **C.** Magnetic resonance imaging scans at the levels of the striatum (B) and the substantia nigra (C). DA, dopamine; Enk, enkephalin; GABA, γ-aminobutyric acid; GPe, globus pallidus – external segment; GPi, globus pallidus – internal segment; IL, intralaminar nuclei of thalamus; SN$_C$, substantia nigra pars compacta; SN$_R$, substantia nigra pars reticulata; SP, substance P; STN, subthalamic nucleus; VA-VL, ventroanterior-ventrolateral nuclei of thalamus.

1.7 What is the substantia nigra?

A dopamine-rich area in the brainstem (*Fig. 1.4*).

The substantia nigra represents a collection of nerve cells found in the midbrain at the top of the structure called the brainstem. These cells are able to manufacture dopamine and they send connecting fibres (axons) up through the brain to the striatum. In the striatum these fibres release dopamine, which works at this site to allow normal movement amongst

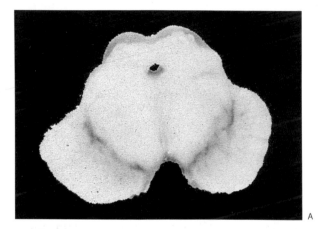

A

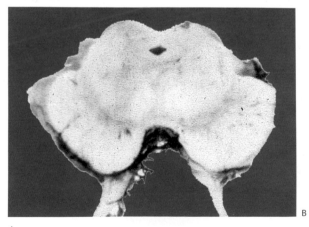

B

▲

Fig. 1.4 Anatomical sections through the midbrain to demonstrate the appearance of the substantia nigra in: **A.** normal people; **B.** Parkinson's disease. Courtesy of Professor Andrew Lees and Dr Tamas Revesz, Institute of Neurology, London.

other things. Dopamine is released from these cells at a background rate and has intermittent pulsatile increases in response to stimulation of the substantia nigra from other brain regions. The substantia nigra cells are also pigmented with melanin, which is where the structure derives its name, 'nigra'. The role of melanin in these cells is not known but may be important in the susceptibility of these neurons to dying in Parkinson's disease.

1.8 What parts of the brain degenerate in Parkinson's disease?

The substantia nigra and a number of other areas.

The major pathway that degenerates in Parkinson's disease is the dopaminergic pathway linking the substantia nigra to the striatum. The loss of this pathway means that the patients have decreasing levels of dopamine, which leads to the major manifestations of the disease and forms the rationale for the treatment with drugs designed to restore normal dopamine levels. Minor deficits in this dopaminergic pathway are not noticeable, but symptoms will result once over half of the dopamine-producing cells are lost. There are also other parts of the nervous system that can be affected in Parkinson's disease; in particular there can be changes within the outer grey matter of the brain, the cortex, which may account for some of the difficulties patients may experience with thinking.

In all the sites of abnormality, there is typically found the pathological microscopic hallmark of Parkinson's disease – the Lewy body.

1.9 What are Lewy bodies?

The pathological hallmark of Parkinson's disease.

Lewy bodies were first described by Joseph Lewy in 1913. They are found within the cytoplasm of cells at sites where nerve cells are dying as a result of the Parkinson's disease process (*Fig. 1.5*). They are therefore most commonly found in the substantia nigra, but are also seen in other sites within the brain. They have recently been found to contain a protein called α-synuclein, and staining for this protein enables Lewy bodies to be easily visualised through a light microscope. The normal function of α-synuclein is not known, but the discovery in the 1990s that a family with an inherited form of Parkinson's disease had a mutation in the gene coding for α-synuclein (*see Q. 1.15*) implies that this protein may be involved in the disease process.

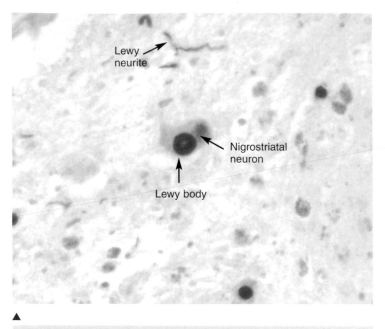

Fig. 1.5 The microscopic appearance of a Lewy body present within the cytoplasm of a surviving nigral cell from a patient who suffered from Parkinson's disease. Courtesy of Dr M G Spillantini, University of Cambridge.

1.10 How common is Parkinson's disease?

The prevalence is about 1 in 1000 individuals.

Parkinson's disease is a common neurological problem affecting about 1 in 1000 people, although this rises to about 1% of the population aged over 55. From prevalence surveys, it seems that the frequency of Parkinson's disease continues to increase even in the very elderly (*Fig. 1.6*), although symptoms of PD may be confused with other disorders in this age group.

In the UK there are approximately 120 000 people with parkinsonism.

1.11 Does Parkinson's disease affect men and women equally?

Yes.

Parkinson's disease appears to affect men slightly more than women, although overall the prevalence (total number of cases) and incidence (number of new cases each year) of the disease are fairly similar in the two sexes.

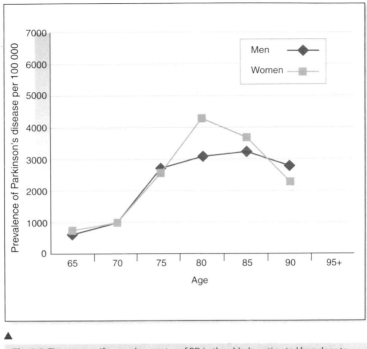

▲

Fig. 1.6 The age-specific prevalence rates of PD in the elderly, estimated by a door-to-door study of PD across five European centres.

1.12   At what age does Parkinson's disease develop?

At any age – but typically between 50–70 years of age.

It is common for Parkinson's disease to develop between the 5th and 8th decade of life, although patients may delay presenting to their doctor for some years. Parkinson's disease can, however, arise at any age, and it is important to consider the diagnosis in patients of any age with typical symptoms of the disease. However, in young patients with PD, it is much more likely that the disease is due to an inherited genetic defect (*see Q. 1.15*). It is also true to say that it is difficult to diagnose Parkinson's disease in the more elderly patient, as many of its features, particularly slowing up or stooping, are not uncommon in this population of patients.

1.13   Is Parkinson's disease found worldwide?

Yes.

Parkinson's disease is found throughout the world, with no obvious major changes in incidence and prevalence across the globe, although lower rates have been described in Africa and China. There are isolated clusters of PD, perhaps the best known being that which occurs in Guam. The reason for this clustering is not clear, but has led to a large amount of work investigating the diet of the people who live on this island. The type of Parkinson's disease which the Guam inhabitants develop is rather different from that seen in the more typical patient and is often associated with other neurological problems, such as dementia and motor neuron disease.

Early surveys in PD suggested that the prevalence of the disorder was higher in whites compared to Asians or blacks but these findings have not been replicated in a more recent door-to-door survey in Mississippi. Blacks and whites living under similar environmental conditions had virtually the same prevalence ratios of PD.

1.14 What causes Parkinson's disease?

Unknown.

> The cause of Parkinson's disease is unknown. There are a large number of theories that have been put forward to explain this condition, but none of them has been substantiated. These various hypotheses include the possibility that Parkinson's disease is due to a genetic abnormality, or occurs as a result of a viral infection, or the result of some environmental toxin, or a combination of environmental and genetic factors. How these putative risk factors might lead to selective death of the dopamine-containing nerve cells of the substantia nigra is also not understood. However, it is becoming increasingly likely that the disease results from multiple *interacting* risk factors, both genetic and environmental. Variation in these risk factors and interactions between them probably explain the variable symptoms observed from one patient to the next (*see Qs 1.23 and 1.24*).

1.15 Is Parkinson's disease inherited?

Very rarely.

There are a few rare families in which Parkinson's disease is inherited because of a clear genetic defect. Attempts to identify the exact position and functions of these genes are ongoing and may be important in advancing our understanding of the disease process in the much more common sporadic form of the disease. Abnormalities at seven possible sites across the genome have been linked with inherited forms of the disease, and these are described in Table 1.2. Most of these abnormal genes are inherited dominantly so that PD symptoms are observed in each generation, with each new family member having a 50% risk of carrying the abnormal gene.

TABLE 1.2 All of the genes/loci currently known to cause
Parkinson's disease within specific families

Mutation name	Chromosome position	Name of gene	Protein function	Mode of inheritance
PARK 1	4q21-22	α-synuclein	Unknown	Autosomal dominant
PARK 2	6q25-27	Parkin	Degradation of intracellular proteins	Autosomal recessive
PARK 3	2p13	Unidentified	Unknown	Autosomal dominant but 40% penetrance
PARK 4	4p14-15	Unidentified	Unknown	Autosomal dominant
PARK 5	4p	UCH-L1	Degradation of intracellular proteins	Autosomal dominant
PARK 6	1p35-36	Unidentified	Unknown	Autosomal recessive
PARK 7	1p36	Unidentified	Unknown	Autosomal recessive
PARK 8	12p11-q12	Unidentified	Unknown	Autosomal dominant

The *PARK2* gene known as 'parkin' is inherited in a recessive fashion.
Patients within such families can only develop the disease if the 'parkin'
gene from both parents is inherited.

Families with these inherited forms of PD often have slightly atypical
disease features in that the patients are often younger than normal and have
unusual responses to therapy. It must be emphasised that these families
with inherited forms of PD are extremely rare. Their importance, however,
should not be underestimated because identifying genetic defects within
them may help elucidate factors that could be important in the genesis of
sporadic PD.

1.16 If a patient has a relative with Parkinson's disease, does that imply the patient has an inherited form of the condition?

No.

As Parkinson's disease is relatively common, it is expected by chance
that many people will have an affected family member. It is therefore not
unusual for patients to have at least one other person in the family with this

condition. Furthermore, because of the difficulty in diagnosing the condition, it is possible that there are patients who think that they have a relative with the condition, who turn out to have some other disorder such as an essential tremor (*see Q. 10.15*).

Patients who develop symptoms of PD at an unusually young age are more likely to have developed the disease through inheriting an abnormal gene, and in these cases, a positive family history may be more relevant (*see Qs 1.15 and 10.12*).

1.17 What is the evidence that Parkinson's disease is due to an environmental toxin?

Limited.

The possibility that Parkinson's disease might be caused by an environmental toxin started when a group of heroin addicts in California in the early 1980s accidentally managed to inject themselves with a toxin called MPTP. This toxin seemed to selectively damage the dopamine cells within the nigrostriatal system, leading to Parkinsonism. These patients responded to therapy, although this was often short lived because of drug-induced side-effects. This toxin was then shown experimentally to induce parkinsonism in a range of animals.

The toxin appeared to have some structural similarities to compounds used in insecticides and it was therefore hypothesised that insecticides may be the cause of Parkinson's disease. A number of studies were therefore undertaken in which the incidence of Parkinson's disease in the countryside, was compared to that found in the city. These studies suggested that PD was slightly more common in the countryside than in the city, but the effect was small and thus the notion that Parkinson's disease is due to an environmental toxin has never truly been substantiated. There has been a small resurgence in interest in pesticides as a possible cause for PD following the recent publication of a report in which the intravenous administration of 'rotenone', a frequently used pesticide, produced features of PD in mice. Furthermore, these mice not only had motor symptoms but also had pathological inclusions similar to Lewy bodies within nigral neurons at post-mortem.

1.18 Is Parkinson's disease the result of a viral infection?

Probably not.

Parkinsonism can occasionally be seen as the consequence of a viral infection of the brain (*see also Q. 10.13*). In the 1920s there was an epidemic of encephalitis lethargica, a curious infection of the brain for which no obvious infective agent was ever found. Significant numbers of these patients developed parkinsonism following this illness and it was therefore hypothesised that all cases of Parkinson's disease could be due to some form of viral infection, perhaps early in life. The incidence of PD has, however, remained constant across time, which argues against a single epidemic viral agent with variable penetrance. Furthermore, post-encephalitic parkinsonism is characterised pathologically by the presence of neurofibrillary tangles in the substantia nigra rather than Lewy bodies. Finally, extensive searches for viral agents have been undertaken in patients with PD, but no single viral agent has ever consistently been found.

1.19   Does smoking cause Parkinson's disease?

No. It is possibly protective.

There is now good evidence from a large number of studies that smoking cigarettes seems to be associated with a lower risk for Parkinson's disease. The reason for this is not clear but the association seems to be genuine rather than due to biased studies or selective mortality in smokers. A recent study also suggests that the protection from PD afforded to smokers is limited to patients carrying a particular gene, and patients not carrying this gene carry an increased risk for PD if they smoke. In any event, it must be stressed that the benefits from not smoking far outweigh any protective value that smoking may have in the genesis of Parkinson's disease.

1.20   Does head trauma cause Parkinson's disease?

Occasionally, if repetitive.

It is unusual to develop Parkinson's disease after a single blow to the head, but repeated chronic injuries to the head can lead to the production of a parkinsonian syndrome. This is perhaps best illustrated in boxers who developed a condition called 'dementia pugilistica' in which repeated head trauma leads to shearing of the nerve fibres from the substantia nigra to the striatum.

Previous epidemiological studies have shown an association between Parkinson's disease and head trauma, although it remains extremely difficult to know how relevant a previous head injury is for an individual presenting with symptoms of PD. When asked, patients with neurological disease often recall a history of head trauma, but this may be due to a recall bias, i.e. patients who have problems relating to their brain tend to remember and attach significance to head injuries to a much greater extent than do neurologically normal people. It is therefore impossible to know whether head trauma truly occurs more frequently in people who go on to develop Parkinson's disease or whether they are simply remembering it more frequently.

1.21 Is Parkinson's disease simply a more rapidly progressive ageing process?

No.

Whilst Parkinson's disease tends to occur more frequently the older you get, it is not simply an accelerated loss of the dopamine cells in the brain. There is now good evidence, from comparing the pathology of brains of patients with Parkinson's disease with brains of people of a similar age, which shows that the loss of dopamine cells that occurs with age is of a very different pattern from that seen in Parkinson's disease. In addition, Lewy bodies are only seen in a small minority of neurologically normal elderly people, at post-mortem.

1.22 How long does it take to develop Parkinson's disease?

Unknown. Probably several years.

It is clear from a number of studies that in order for patients to present with Parkinson's disease they have had to lose at least half of the normal number of dopamine cells in their substantia nigra. However, it is currently unresolved as to how quickly this loss of cells occurs. There is some recent evidence using PET scanning to assess dopamine levels in the living brain, that patients developing Parkinson's disease normally start to lose the cells 5–10 years before they present clinically. It is also entirely possible that different patients may lose their dopamine-producing cells at different rates depending on their age of onset (*see Qs 1.23 and 1.24*).

1.23 Does Parkinson's disease present in any one way?

No.

There are multiple ways in which Parkinson's disease can present, which coupled with the subtle deficits seen early on, can make it extremely difficult to diagnose in the early stages. Many patients may be completely undisturbed by their symptoms and corroborative accounts from family members may be required to fully ascertain the extent and breadth of symptoms and signs. It is also highly probable that there are different types of Parkinson's disease, which may have different causes, different prognoses, and respond to treatments in different ways.

1.24 What are the different types of Parkinson's disease?

Unresolved, but probably a more benign tremor form of the disease exists.

Although there is no consensus on what constitutes the different subtypes of Parkinson's disease, there is some evidence that there is a tremor-dominant form of the condition which tends to run a much more benign course, in contrast to the more rigid/akinetic form of the condition, in which tremor is much less of a feature and the patients tend to progress more quickly. It is likely that the differing clinical forms of PD are related to differing underlying pathological processes, and there is some evidence that the substantia nigra has a different regional pattern of cell loss in these different subtypes of patients.

There is also additional evidence that the rate of loss of nigral neurons is slower in PD patients carrying the *PARK2* gene ('parkin'), although the process of cell loss must have started earlier to account for the younger age at presentation. Further genetic, epidemiological and pathophysiological studies will all be required to completely understand the processes that underlie the differing types of PD.

Many patients do not clearly fall into either of the two main clinical categories (tremor dominant; rigid/akinetic), which relates to the fact that this subdivision is probably far too simplistic.

1.25   How can anyone be certain that a patient has Parkinson's disease?

Ultimately this can only be done at post-mortem.

Although doctors can ultimately be confident that patients have Parkinson's disease clinically, unfortunately the only way one can be certain is through post-mortem analysis of the brain, with the demonstration of Lewy bodies at specific sites within it, particularly the substantia nigra. Currently, clinical diagnoses of PD are correct in about 80% of cases. The clinical features listed in Box 1.1 increase the specificity for the diagnosis.

In some specialist centres there are special scans that can be done of the brain to look at dopamine within it, these scans are called positron-emission tomography scans or PET scans (*see Q. 4.6*). These can be very helpful in diagnosing Parkinson's disease in life, but because such few scanners exist, they are mainly used for research purposes, and so are rarely of use for most patients with Parkinson's disease.

BOX 1.1 Clinical features supporting the diagnosis of PD

■ Asymmetric onset
■ Dominant motor symptoms
■ Absence of other neurological or cognitive deficits
■ Good response to dopamine therapy

1.26   What are the stages of Parkinson's disease?

There are five stages from presymptomatic to palliative (*Fig. 1.7*).

It is estimated that there is a presymptomatic phase of approximately 5 years during which time nigral neurons are being lost but the number of remaining neurons is sufficient to prevent the onset of overt symptoms. As

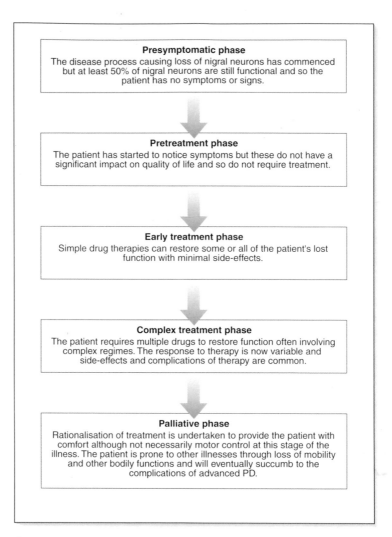

Fig. 1.7 Figure to demonstrate the progression of Parkinson's disease. The duration of each phase is highly variable from one person to the next.

the disease progresses, a critical threshold for the development of symptoms is reached, which may or may not lead to the patient presenting to his or her doctor. Symptoms at this stage may be very mild and may not require treatment. The patient will, however, eventually enter a phase where drug treatment is required – the early treatment phase – and drug therapy is usually straightforward at this stage. This phase of the illness tends to last on average for 3–10 years. At the conclusion of this phase, the patient develops complications of drug therapy and this signifies the onset of the complex treatment phase, where complex regimes of drugs are employed with side-effects and drug-induced complications. Finally, a palliative phase is entered where the comfort rather than the motor control of the patient is paramount.

Margaret Hoehn and Melvin Yahr published a detailed description of the progression of PD in the 1960s, and a numerical scale based on their description has been widely used since then. It is summarised in Box 1.2.

Schwab & England developed a further scale used to quantify the relative stages of PD (*Box 1.3*). This scale is based on an individual's ability to perform household chores and can be difficult to use in some patients who have never performed housework.

BOX 1.2 The modified Hoehn and Yahr scale (Hoehn & Yahr 1967, reproduced by permission of Professor Stanley Fahn)

Stage 0   = No signs of disease.
Stage 1   = Unilateral disease.
Stage 1.5 = Unilateral plus axial involvement.
Stage 2   = Bilateral disease, without any impairment of balance.
Stage 2.5 = Mild bilateral disease, with recovery of balance on being pulled gently backwards (pull test).
Stage 3   = Mild to moderate bilateral disease; some postural instability (i.e. abnormal pull test); physically independent.
Stage 4   = Severe disability; still able to walk or stand unassisted.
Stage 5   = Wheelchair bound or bedridden unless aided.

BOX 1.3 The Schwab & England activities of daily living scale (reproduced by permission of Professor Stanley Fahn)

100% = Completely independent. Able to do all chores without slowness, difficulty or impairment. Essentially normal. Unaware of any difficulty.

90% = Completely independent. Able to do all chores with some degree of slowness, difficulty and impairment. Might take twice as long. Beginning to be aware of difficulty.

80% = Completely independent in most chores. Takes twice as long. Conscious of difficulty and slowness.

70% = Not completely independent. More difficulty with some chores. Three to four times as long in some. Must spend a large part of the day with chores.

60% = Some dependency. Can do most chores, but exceedingly slowly and with much effort and errors. Some tasks are impossible.

50% = More dependent. Help with half of their daily activities, slower, etc. Difficulty with everything.

40% = Very dependent. Can assist with all chores, but few alone.

30% = With effort, now and then does a few chores alone or begins alone. Much help needed.

20% = Nothing alone. Can be a slight help with some chores. Severe invalid.

10% = Totally dependent, helpless. Complete invalid.

0% = Vegetative functions such as swallowing, bladder and bowel functions are not functioning. Bedridden.

PQ PATIENT QUESTIONS

What caused my Parkinson's disease?

No-one is able to tell you for certain what caused your Parkinson's disease.
The little that we know at the moment suggests that there is a whole range of
environmental exposures that might lead to an increased risk of developing
Parkinson's disease. Some people with Parkinson's disease, however, have
never encountered any of these exposures and many people who do
encounter these risks *do not* go on to develop Parkinson's disease.

It is also possible that we all carry a certain risk for Parkinson's disease in
our genes and only people who have these 'elevated risk' genes and then also
become exposed to environmental risks go on to develop this disorder.
Research is being done to find out more about these possible Parkinson's
disease risk genes and the environmental exposures that might be to blame.

Could pesticides have caused my Parkinson's disease?

Both herbicides and insecticides have been previously thought to be possible
causes of Parkinson's disease. Not all research studies have, however,
confirmed this. If you have had long-term exposure to these types of
chemicals, it is indeed possible that they have contributed to you developing
the disease. At the same time, it is also possible that you might have
developed Parkinson's disease even without being exposed to pesticide
chemicals. Until we know more about the level of risk that may be due to
pesticides, there is no way of knowing whether these chemicals in any way
caused your disease. (*See also Qs 1.17 and 9.22.*)

Are my children at risk of Parkinson's disease?

Just because you have developed symptoms of Parkinson's disease, this does
not mean that your children are at increased risk. Very rarely, Parkinson's
disease can run in families because of an abnormal gene being passed on
from generation to generation. The majority of people with Parkinson's
disease, however, do not carry these abnormal genes, and unless you have
several other close relatives with Parkinson's disease, there is no reason to
think that you have one of these genes. Moreover, the majority of patients
who do have one of these inherited forms of Parkinson's disease develop
symptoms at a particularly young age, typically before the age of 30. Many
individuals with Parkinson's disease are aware of another family member
with symptoms or a diagnosis of this condition, but unless the disease is
consistently occurring in successive generations, it is very unlikely that your
children are at a significantly elevated risk.

Recognising a patient with Parkinson's disease: history and examination

2

2.1 Can I spot Parkinson's disease as the patient walks into the room?

Sometimes yes.

The first impression of a Parkinson's disease patient walking into the consultation room might in some cases suggest the diagnosis. A lack of facial expression (*hypomimia*) may be confused with depression, but when seen together with reduced arm swing on walking, a characteristic stooping gait, or resting tremor, a diagnosis of PD should always be considered. The majority of patients, however, do not have very obvious signs at the onset of their disease, and a careful history and neurological examination are necessary. In advanced disease, a patient's posture and gait tend to reveal the diagnosis before the patient has even sat down.

2.2 What are the classical features of Parkinson's disease?

Resting tremor, slowness of movement and an expressionless face.

The classical features of Parkinson's disease include an asymmetric resting, *pill rolling tremor*, which typically affects the hand, although it can spread to involve the leg and jaw. It rarely involves the head, or the voice. In addition, patients complain of a slowness of moving, such that they often have difficulty getting going or initiating a movement; this is termed *bradykinesia* or *akinesia*. In addition, the arms on moving them are somewhat stiffer than normal and this is called *rigidity*.

2.3 What are the most common presenting complaints of Parkinson's disease patients?

Often non-specific vague symptoms.

Most patients with Parkinson's disease present with one of a number of possible complaints:

- a resting tremor affecting one side of the body, typically the hand
- a change in handwriting, such that it becomes smaller or more scribbly
- a loss of dexterity of a hand, for example doing up buttons or shoelaces, or when using a knife and fork
- dragging of the leg when walking
- a general slowing up, often with aching of the muscles
- the voice becoming quieter
- loss of facial expression
- a frozen shoulder
- reduced exercise tolerance.

2.4 Can a history distinguish Parkinson's disease tremor from other causes of tremor?

Occasionally yes.

Differentiating a parkinsonian tremor from a benign essential tremor or a cerebellar tremor can be very difficult (*Table 2.1*). Parkinson's disease tremors almost always start asymmetrically, whereas essential tremor patients tend to have a bilateral tremor, often also affecting the head, lips or chin. About half of the essential tremor patients (*see Q. 10.15*) have a family history of tremor and about half also find that their tremor is relieved following moderate intake of alcohol, which is not the case for PD tremor. Essential tremor patients also tend to present at a younger age than patients with PD.

TABLE 2.1 Distinguishing PD, essential and cerebellar tremors

	PD tremor	Essential tremor	Cerebellar tremor
Age at onset	Majority age 50–70	Onset age 20–50	Variable
Tremor type	Resting > action Asymmetric	Action > resting Symmetrical	Intention
Aggravating/ relieving factors	Worse with anxiety	Relief with alcohol	
Other clues	Bradykinesia	Involvement of head and neck	Ataxia

Although classically described as a rest tremor, many PD patients describe a worsening of their tremor during actions such as drinking from a teacup, or when carrying heavy objects. A tremor occurring exclusively with actions or intention, that completely disappears with rest, may be more suggestive of a cerebellar tremor. The frequency or amplitude of the tremor is rarely helpful in distinguishing the underlying causes.

2.5 What other aspects of the history are important for patients with tremor?

Symptoms of hyperthyroidism or drug exposure.

Tremor is occasionally the presenting complaint of patients with hyperthyroidism. This type of tremor occurs with posture holding more commonly than at rest. Other symptoms such as sweating, palpitations or diarrhoea may provide clues that a tremor is secondary to hyperactive thyroid disease.

Previous or current exposure to drugs that act on the dopaminergic system may be relevant to the development, or the unmasking, of a parkinsonian tremor. Dopamine antagonists such as the neuroleptic agents used in psychiatry, antiemetics such as prochlorperazine (Stemetil) or metoclopramide (Maxolon) may be contributing to a patient's symptoms and attempts should be made to stop or reduce these agents. Drug-induced parkinsonism tends to be largely reversible on stopping the offending drug.

2.6   What is orthostatic tremor?

Tremor of the legs at rest relieved by walking.

Orthostatic tremor is very rare and refers to a tremor that occurs in the legs on standing still. This type of tremor is typically relieved by walking. The cause of this form of tremor is not known, but a few patients may develop symptoms or signs of Parkinson's disease years later. This type of tremor is best treated with clonazepam.

2.7   How is a Parkinson's disease tremor best observed?

Often by distracting the patient with another task.

Patients may not always volunteer that they have a tremor and may focus on other symptoms rather than the tremor during a consultation. Some patients subconsciously hide any tremor by sitting on their hands, or placing their hands in their pockets when in company. Resting tremor is best observed by ensuring that the patient's hand is relaxed, and not touching any other part of the body. Further distracting the patient with either a task requiring the use of the contralateral hand or a request to count backwards aloud can make the Parkinson's disease tremor more apparent.

Attempts to quantify the degree of tremor, bradykinesia and rigidity in a patient with PD should use the standard, validated Unified Parkinson's Disease Rating Scale (UPDRS). This is reproduced in Appendix 1.

2.8   How can bradykinesia be demonstrated in the hand or foot?

By getting the patient to perform repetitive movements.

Asking the patient to perform finger taps with thumb and index finger can reveal both low frequency and small amplitude of movements, which progressively become slower and smaller with repetition. The standard method used to assess bradykinesia is to count how many finger taps can be completed in a 5-second period, and observe for the premature development of decreasing speed and amplitude. Hand bradykinesia is also often made obvious by asking a patient to quickly and repetitively open and close the hand. It should be remembered, however, that an inability to perform rapid finger taps or hand opening and closing is not specifically a sign of bradykinesia due to Parkinson's disease. A range of neurological disorders affecting movement and muscles as well as musculoskeletal problems can lead to difficulties performing these simple tasks.

A patient with symptoms affecting the leg will also often have difficulty in performing regular, repetitive foot taps. Loss in timing or amplitude of foot tapping is often seen in PD.

2.9 Are there any other causes of bradykinesia?

Yes.

In addition to Parkinson's disease, any of the causes of secondary parkinsonism or Parkinson-plus diseases can present with bradykinesia (*see Table 10.1*). Bradykinesia can also occur in other neurodegenerative basal ganglia diseases such as Huntington's disease; however, other symptoms and signs tend to dominate the clinical picture in these disorders. Bradykinesia can also be seen in some psychiatric conditions such as depression. Pain or stiffness due to arthritis, or excessive muscle spasms may sometimes lead to slowed movements that can be confused with bradykinesia due to PD.

2.10 What is cogwheeling?

The ratchet feel of increased tone in a limb with tremor.

Cogwheel rigidity can be felt during assessment of the patient's muscle tone. The coexistence of tremor with increased resistance to passive movements can be felt as a ratchet-like sensation known as cogwheeling. This is most easily detected by passively rotating the patient's wrist, and may be made more obvious by asking the patient to perform a task with the contralateral limb. The phenomenon of unintentional muscle contraction accompanying contraction of another group of muscles is known as '*synkinesis*'. Increased tone may also be noted in the patient's other limb joints or neck.

2.11 What other causes are there of increased muscle tone?

Many, including spasticity.

Increased muscle tone is not always due to rigidity (*Box 2.1*). Rigidity affects flexor and extensor muscles equally and should be distinguished from spasticity, which tends to affect predominantly arm flexors and leg extensors. Spasticity is also usually associated with brisk reflexes and even

---

BOX 2.1 The causes of increased muscle tone

- Extrapyramidal diseases such as PD
- Spasticity
- Gegenhalten
- Pain
- Anxiety (failure to relax)
- Stiff man syndrome (rare)

clonus, and occurs following damage to the descending motor pathways from the brain to the spinal cord. An increase in muscle tone known as *gegenhalten* occurs following damage to the frontal lobes and leads to increase in tone whenever the patient attempts to relax the limb. Increased tone due to gegenhalten disappears when a patient is sufficiently distracted. An involuntary increase in muscle tone may occur as a protective response to muscle or joint injuries.

Parkinson's disease patients may exhibit either 'lead pipe rigidity' where resistance to passive movement is fairly even throughout the movement or 'cogwheel rigidity' as described above (*see Q. 2.10*). Cogwheeling without an increase in tone can also be felt in patients with benign essential tremor.

2.12 Does a patient have to have all of the classical features to have Parkinson's disease?

No.

> It is not uncommon for patients with Parkinson's disease to present with only one or two out of the classical features of PD (*see Q. 2.2*). Indeed some patients with pathologically proven PD never show all of the features of PD. This can make the diagnosis difficult in the first instance. A thorough history and examination may reveal the patient to have other symptoms that aid in the diagnosis of PD.

2.13 What is the characteristic gait disturbance of Parkinson's disease?

A stooped posture with shuffling gait and reduced arm swing.

Abnormalities in walking and gait are very common at all stages of the disease. The patient often has a shuffling gait and may be slightly hunched and bent at the knees. The speed of walking is often slowed, and this may be more noticeable to the patient's spouse who may need to wait for the patient while they are walking together. Reduction in the natural arm swing in the affected arm is also characteristic of Parkinson's disease. As the disease progresses, not only do these abnormalities become more prominent but patients also discover that they become frozen to the spot and are unable to initiate walking (*see Q. 7.5*). This is often precipitated by doorways or moving through other enclosed spaces. Freezing episodes can be overcome by simple manoeuvres such as imagining stepping over an object, and in the early stages often respond reasonably well to drug treatment.

2.14 What is a festinant gait?

Short shuffling steps.

Festination is derived from the Latin verb for hurrying and describes the short shuffling steps characteristically seen in patients with Parkinson's disease. They appear to be continually trying to catch up with themselves.

2.15 What causes Parkinson's disease patients to fall?

There are many causes.

Falls are a leading cause of morbidity and mortality in the elderly population and are especially common among sufferers of Parkinson's disease. Table 2.2 outlines the common causes of falls among PD patients.

TABLE 2.2 Common causes of falling in Parkinson's disease

Cause of falling	Clues from the history and examination	Further discussion and treatment options
Parkinson's disease causing postural instability	Falls occurring when turning, getting out of a chair, or bending over. Abnormal 'pull test'*	Questions 2.30, 9.6
Parkinson's disease causing postural hypotension	Falls occurring after standing, often accompanied by a sensation of light-headedness	Question 6.6
Parkinson's disease causing freezing and festination	Patients describe hesitation on starting, or attempting to turn. Festinant patients try to 'keep up' with their upper body	Questions 7.5, 7.6, 9.7
L-dopa-induced dyskinesia	Loss of balance due to involuntary movements (relatively uncommon)	Questions 7.11, 7.12
Local environmental factors	Tripping up over small objects on the floor, poor lighting, unsafe stairways poorly fitting or non-supportive footwear. Best assessed during domiciliary visit	Question 9.4
Coexisting neurological disorder	Features of stroke, epilepsy, cervical or lumbar spine problems or sensory deficits. The Parkinson-plus disorders	Chapter 10
Other medical disorder	Features of arthritis, cardiac disease, impaired vision, alcohol abuse, and other causes	

* The pull test: After adequate explanation and warning, postural reflex impairment can be assessed by gently pulling backwards a patient who is standing with the feet slightly apart.

Falls are more likely to occur in patients with Parkinson-plus disorders, and these diagnoses should be considered when falls are a prominent feature early during the disease course (*see Ch. 10*).

2.16 Are the eyes affected in Parkinson's disease?

Rarely, and normally with respect to opening and closing.

Most patients with Parkinson's disease do not experience any problems with their eyes. In particular, the ability to see should not be affected by this condition. However, some patients experience difficulty with controlling the opening and shutting of their eyelids, such that some of them experience prolonged eyelid shutting for no apparent reason. This is termed *apraxia* of eyelid opening and closing. It can often be relieved by simply rubbing the eyelid. Severe eyelid apraxia is more suggestive of a Parkinson-plus syndrome, and occasionally this may require treatment with botulinum toxin injections with or without minor surgical elevation procedures to the eyelids.

Patients with glaucoma should not be given anticholinergic drugs for their PD.

2.17 Is sleep affected in Parkinson's disease?

Yes, normally because of insufficient treatment.

There are multiple possible causes of disturbed sleep at night in patients with Parkinson's disease, and these are summarised in Table 2.3. The impact of PD or nocturnal insomnia on increasing sleepiness during the day can be most reliably quantified using the Epworth sleepiness scale, which is reproduced in Figure 2.1. Treatments of disturbed sleep are discussed in Chapter 6 (*Q. 6.7*).

As a secondary effect of disturbed sleep at night, patients can also suffer from excessive daytime drowsiness, or more rarely from 'sleep attacks' during the day. These attacks occur more frequently in men and in advanced PD, and have been associated with motor vehicle accidents. In addition there has been recent interest in the possibility that these may be provoked by dopaminergic medication (*see also Q. 5.10*). Patients who are prone to these attacks should obviously be told not to drive.

2.18 Is smell affected in Parkinson's disease?

Usually yes, but not typically to a symptomatic level.

The ability to smell is not usually abnormal in patients with Parkinson's disease, although if rigorously tested, disturbances in the function of the olfactory system can be detected early on in the condition. However, most patients are not aware of this abnormality and its use in terms of diagnosis

---

TABLE 2.3 Causes of disturbed sleep in Parkinson's disease

Causes of disturbed sleep	Commonly due to
Insomnia	Difficulty turning over in bed Persistent tremor keeping patient awake L-dopa-induced dyskinesias Depression Anxiety Dopaminergic medication causing a state of overexcitement
Nightmares	Rapid eye movement sleep behaviour disorder (RSBD)* Dopaminergic medication Hallucinations
Restless legs	Restless legs syndrome† Iron deficiency
Nocturia	Bladder instability Prostatism Urinary infections
Dementia	Confusion Drug therapy

* REM sleep behaviour disorder is particularly common in PD. It is characterised by complex movements occurring during dreaming in REM sleep. Injuries can occur both to patients and their partners as a result of these movements. Polysomnography shows loss of the muscle relaxation which normally occurs during REM sleep and is necessary to confirm the diagnosis, which responds well to treatment.

†Restless legs syndrome occurs in about 6% of the normal adult population, and about 20% of PD patients. Patients experience uncomfortable legs with inactivity which is temporarily relieved by moving the limbs.

---

is unresolved. Loss of the sense of smell may also be a feature of other conditions such as Alzheimer's disease although it is not usually seen in the Parkinson-plus disorders. Of course, the commonest cause for a loss of smell relates to local inflammation/infection in the nasal cavities.

2.19 Is speech affected in Parkinson's disease?

Yes, it is typically quiet and mumbling.

Most patients with Parkinson's disease experience some difficulty with speech. In the first instance this is often manifest as low speech volume (hypophonia), and patients may have problems raising the voice. This can become more marked as the disease progresses, such that some patients later on in the disease can scarcely be heard to talk. In addition, the difficulty in initiating movements in the arms and in the legs with walking,

Epworth sleepiness scale

Name

Today's date

Your age (years)

Your sex (male = M female = F)

How likely are you to doze off or fall asleep in the following situations, in contrast to just feeling tired? This refers to your usual way of life in recent times.
Even if you have not done some of these things recently try to work out how they would have affected you.
Use the following scale to choose the *most appropriate number* for each situation:

0 - would *never* doze
1 - *slight* chance of dozing
2 - *moderate* chance of dozing
3 - *high* chance of dozing

It is important that you answer each question as best you can.

Situation   **Chance of dozing**

Sitting and reading

Watching TV

Sitting, inactive in a public place (e.g. a theatre or a meeting)

As a passenger in a car for an hour without a break

Lying down to rest in the afternoon when circumstances permit

Sitting and talking to someone

Sitting quietly after lunch without alcohol

In a car while stopped for a few minutes in the traffic

Thank you for your cooperation   Total

* Scores of >10 are consistent with excessive daytime sleepiness

▲

Fig. 2.1 The Epworth sleepiness scale. Reproduced with permission of Professor Murray W Johns.

can also be seen with speech; therefore patients can present with great difficulty in expressing themselves and getting their words out. This is often extremely frustrating for them, as the people they are conversing with will tend to complete their sentences for them.

2.20 Is dribbling of saliva a feature of Parkinson's disease?

Yes.

One of the early features of Parkinson's disease can be the slowness of muscle contraction within the perioral muscles leading to the drooling of saliva out of the corner of the mouth. Initially, this symptom may only be noticed because the patient's pillow is slightly damp in the mornings and requires no intervention other than an occasional tissue. As the disease progresses some people develop excessive drooling, which can lead to great embarrassment and may require drug treatment (*see Q. 6.2*).

2.21 Is swallowing affected in Parkinson's disease?

Only usually in advanced disease.

In advanced disease, Parkinson's disease can also progress to involve the muscles of the pharynx, leading to difficulties in swallowing that may increase the problem of saliva dribbling. Ultimately swallowing can be so severely affected as to make treatment with oral drugs extremely difficult, especially in 'off' periods, and other routes of drug administration may need to be considered, e.g. subcutaneous apomorphine injections (*see Qs 7.17 and 7.18*). In such circumstances, dietary modifications and the possibility of percutaneous endoscopic gastrostomy (PEG) may be required to prevent excessive weight loss (*see also Q. 9.11*).

2.22 Is abnormal sweating a feature of Parkinson's disease?

On occasions, but it is unusual.

An increase in sweating can be seen in patients with established Parkinson's disease, both as a response to treatment and more commonly occurring as the treatment wears off. It is likely that dopamine systems play a role in thermoregulation; however, the precise mechanisms are not entirely clear. Excessive sweating in PD may also have other causes such as thyrotoxicosis or a postmenopausal state.

Excessive secretion of oil by sebaceous glands with seborrhoea of the head, face, and neck is also common in PD. Treatment of sweating and seborrhoea is discussed in Chapter 6 (*Q. 6.3*).

2.23 Do Parkinson's disease patients experience numbness or tingling in their arms or legs?

No, although sensory symptoms can be due to rigidity.

Patients with Parkinson's disease do not commonly experience any numbness or tingling in their arms or legs, and when it is a prominent feature other causes should be excluded. However, it is very common for patients with PD to complain of stiffness and aching in their muscles, which presumably relates to the rigidity and inability to activate them.

2.24   Is the bladder affected in Parkinson's disease?

Yes, but only to a minor extent.

One of the problems in the diagnosis of Parkinson's disease is that because it affects an elderly population, other disease processes can complicate the clinical situation. It is therefore not uncommon for male patients with PD to have problems with their prostate gland, which can affect their ability to pass water. Furthermore, patients with PD can experience slight bladder disturbance in that the bladder can feel slightly irritable such that the need to pass water can be there for most of the time and be an irritation. However, if bladder disturbances are a very dominant feature of the condition then other causes should be thought of, including local problems within the bladder, such as infection or stones, problems in the lower spine, such as a cauda equina lesion, or one of the Parkinson-plus conditions, especially multiple system atrophy (*see Ch. 10*).

2.25   What happens to bowel function in Parkinson's disease?

Constipation.

Constipation is a very common feature of Parkinson's disease and probably relates to the fact that the disease process can affect the nerves within the gut. Indeed Lewy bodies have been seen in degenerating neurons in the myenteric plexus of the colon of PD patients. It has even been hypothesised that people with infrequent bowel habits are at increased risk of subsequently developing PD. Irrespective of this, it is extremely common for people with PD to have marked problems with constipation, which often does not respond to the usual treatments for PD. These patients often therefore require increased dietary fibre, laxatives or gut stimulants (*see Q. 6.4.*).

2.26   Is postural hypotension a feature of Parkinson's disease?

Yes, but rarely a major feature.

Everybody feels faint or dizzy when they stand up, if they do it quickly enough. This is because the blood pressure takes a while to return to normal, and there is a slight pooling of blood in the feet, with insufficient quantities reaching the brain. In Parkinson's disease there is often mild disturbance of the autonomic nerves, controlling the blood pressure such that this dizziness on standing can be more prominent. Furthermore, this can be made worse by some of the drug treatments which can also affect this part of the nervous system. It is therefore not uncommon for people with PD to feel, or be more prone to feeling, faint on standing quickly. However, if this is the dominant feature of the illness then it raises suspicion that the patient may actually have a Parkinson-plus condition such as multiple system atrophy (*see Ch. 10*).

2.27 What other aspects of the history are important?

Relevant family history and the social situation of the patient.

A family history of Parkinson's disease or other neurological condition can help in diagnosing atypical forms of PD, although patients must be reassured that a family history of the disease does not necessarily imply an inherited risk.

During serial consultations, time should also be spent on identifying the extent of the social support that an individual has, and the extent to which individuals are able to cope with their symptoms. Symptoms of PD may have a profound impact on domestic and family life, in addition to work and social activities. These issues are discussed further in Chapter 9.

2.28 What extra symptoms may be described by a patient already on drug treatment?

The development of involuntary movements, nausea and postural hypotension.

The commonest abnormality that people experience when they take treatment for Parkinson's disease is abnormal movements. These movements often occur after a number of years of taking medication and consist of *dance-like rapid movements* of the arms and legs, normally 30 minutes to an hour after taking the medication. These movements are known as dyskinesias and, although completely dissimilar to other features of PD, do not normally cause diagnostic confusion, since most patients with dyskinesias have been diagnosed with PD and warned about the risk of these movements years earlier (*see Q. 7.11*). Dyskinesias can be extremely severe and cause patients to fall out of chairs, in addition to causing distress to carers and family members. Anti-parkinsonian drugs can also, however, cause *fixed posturing* of the arms or legs known as dystonias, which are another type of dyskinesia and can be extremely painful. These most frequently occur early in the morning before a patient has had the first dose of medication, but can also occur during periods of peak drug levels.

In these situations some patients elect to radically reduce their amounts of treatment, as they find these abnormal movements more disabling and painful than the actual disease itself.

2.29 What is a positive glabellar tap sign?

A sustained blink response to tapping between the eyes.

The glabellar area is located between the eyes and is innervated by the trigeminal nerve. Light tapping of this region with a finger leads to a blink response in normal people; however, this blink response tends to diminish following repetitive tapping. Some patients with Parkinson's disease cannot suppress a blink each time the region is tapped, i.e. have a sustained blink response. This is known as the 'positive glabellar tap sign'. This sign, however, is not a finding specific to PD, nor is it seen in all PD patients and therefore is of limited diagnostic value.

2.30 What happens to a patient's reflexes in Parkinson's disease?

They remain normal in the limbs, but abnormal postural reflexes are common.

The tendon reflexes are not affected in Parkinson's disease, and if absent or pathologically brisk raise the suspicion of another diagnosis, or a second disease process. Postural reflexes, however, are frequently impaired as the disease progresses, which explains the tendency for some patients to fall. The pull test (*see Table 2.2* – footnote) can be used to assess postural reflex impairment.

PQ PATIENT QUESTIONS

Could my symptoms be due to a trapped nerve?

Nerves supplying the muscles of the arms and legs leave the spinal cord and pass through gaps between the vertebrae. Wear and tear, or injuries to the vertebrae can lead to these nerves being compressed or 'trapped'. Patients with trapped nerves are likely to present with pain (similar to sciatica), weakness or muscle wasting as their dominant symptoms. It is very unusual for tremor or muscle stiffness to occur following nerve compression. Even though your symptoms are restricted to one arm, it is very unlikely that there is a mechanical cause for your tremor. It is far more likely that your symptoms are due to Parkinson's disease.

Why does my tremor get worse when I'm anxious?

All people with tremor find that it gets worse during times of stress or anxiety, no matter what the cause. The tremor due to your Parkinson's disease is no exception. If the tremor is particularly bad in certain situations, it may be sensible either to avoid those situations or, if that is not possible, you may want to try a tablet that can lessen anxiety, such as one of the β-blockers called propranolol (*see* Q. 5.29).

Disorders of mood and thinking in Parkinson's disease

3

3.1   Is dementia a feature of Parkinson's disease?

Yes. In about a quarter of cases.

About 25–40% of patients with Parkinson's disease will ultimately develop a dementia. It is unclear at this stage whether patients who develop a dementia represent a distinct disease group separate from standard Parkinson's disease, or whether their condition is part of PD. Many patients will complain that they have impaired memory or are unable to perform mental processes normally, and careful assessment is often required to determine the extent and profile of memory impairments. When cognitive impairment is suspected in an individual with PD, it is important to consider a range of other possible causes as well as depression (see Table 3.1).

The Mini Mental State Examination, samples from which are outlined in Appendix 1, can be used to briefly assess a patient's cognitive function.

TABLE 3.1   Causes of cognitive impairment found in PD patients

Cause of cognitive impairment	Clues to distinguishing cause
Underlying Parkinson's disease pathology	Gradual impairment in memory for recent news and events, with progression of motor features of PD
Depression (pseudo-dementia)	Other biological features of depression such as insomnia and decreased appetite
Dementia of Alzheimer's type	Gradual impairment in anterograde memory, predominantly for time, place and person
Cerebral vascular disease	Stepwise deterioration in cognitive ability along with other non-PD neurological deficits
Parkinson-plus syndrome	Other deficits such as hallucinations, or non-parkinsonian neurological signs
Medications (e.g. trihexyphenidyl (benzhexol), dopaminergic agents)	Newly introduced medication
Other causes, e.g. chronic subdural haematoma	Fluctuating cognitive ability. History of head trauma

3.2   What predicts whether a patient with Parkinson's disease will get dementia?

There are no clear predictors, but it is more common in advanced disease.

Dementia occurring early in the course of the disease is unusual and should raise the suspicion that the patient has dementia with Lewy bodies. It is impossible to predict whether patients will go on to develop a dementia based on their initial symptoms of Parkinson's disease, although there is some suggestion that tremor-dominant patients develop less dementia. In advanced PD, dementia becomes more common, but again its occurrence is not related to either the presence or severity of tremor, stiffness or slowness. Sadly those patients with cognitive impairment have been shown to have a higher prevalence of depression and are more likely to suffer with hallucinations. These features may occur as a secondary consequence of the motor symptoms of PD but it has also been suggested that the underlying neurodegenerative disease process is also the cause of cognitive impairment, depression and hallucinations in PD patients.

3.3   What is dementia with Lewy bodies (DLB)?

An entity with prominent fluctuating cognitive impairments and parkinsonism with large numbers of cortical Lewy bodies.

Dementia with Lewy bodies (DLB) is a common cause of dementia (second only to Alzheimer's dementia). It is now accepted that Lewy bodies can be found throughout the cerebral cortex in both Parkinson's disease and other conditions, but most abundantly in the condition referred to as DLB. In this disease, whilst large numbers of Lewy bodies are found throughout the cerebral cortex, causing the cognitive deficits, the patients also have motor features that may appear identical to those seen in PD. The features of DLB that help to distinguish it from PD are the fluctuation in cognitive state, the relatively rapid deterioration of cognitive performance, and the presence of hallucinations, often all provoked by medication for PD. Most cases of DLB progress to frank dementia within a couple of years of onset. It is currently unclear whether or not DLB and PD represent two distinct conditions or if there is a diffuse spectrum of disease with PD at one end and DLB at the other. Certainly there is evidence that cortical Lewy bodies play some role in the cognitive impairment in both PD and DLB.

3.4   What is the relationship between dementia in Parkinson's disease and other types of dementia?

They relate to each other through their pathological characteristics.

There are many causes of dementia which are now being classified according to their common pathological inclusions. In the context of Parkinson's disease, this is in the form of α-synuclein Lewy bodies, whilst in Parkinson-plus conditions, the inclusions can involve α-synuclein or another protein called tau. As a result, these diseases are sometimes referred to as synucleinopathies or tauopathies (*see Box 3.1*).

BOX 3.1 Diseases associated with abnormal α-synuclein or tau protein

Synucleinopathies
- Lewy body diseases
- Idiopathic Parkinson's disease
- Dementia with Lewy bodies
- Multiple system atrophy (*see Ch. 10*)

Tauopathies
- Alzheimer's disease
- Pick's disease
- Progressive supranuclear palsy
- Corticobasal degeneration
- Frontotemporal dementia and parkinsonism linked to chromosome 17 (FTDP-17)

3.5 Can medications make cognitive impairment in Parkinson's disease worse?

 Yes.

 Medications used in Parkinson's disease may worsen cognitive impairment, especially in those patients where there is already evidence of significant mental impairment. Certain medications are especially prone to causing this, including anticholinergic medications, which can even cause a degree of confusion in cognitively intact elderly patients (even those not progressing to dementia with Lewy bodies). As a rule these should be avoided in patients above the age of 65. The reason for this is that the cholinergic system is important in memory processing and cognition, and the disruption of this system is thought to play a contributory role to the memory deficits seen in Alzheimer's disease. In addition, L-dopa and dopaminergic agents, whilst improving physical symptoms in PD, may also cause a range of cognitive problems ranging from mild disturbances in concentration through to frank confusion and hallucinations.

A patient in whom cognitive impairment is seen following the introduction of a new medication should have the new drug stopped first. When it is not clear which medications are contributing to cognitive impairment, it is wise to stop the anticholinergic therapies first, followed by selegiline, amantadine, dopamine agonists, and COMT inhibitors in that order, prior to lowering the L-dopa dose (*see also Chs 5, 6 and 7*).

3.6 Is cognitive impairment as disabling as the motor impairments of Parkinson's disease?

Yes, if not more so.

Many patients complain that despite coming to terms with the physical aspects of their disease, cognitive impairment is very difficult to cope with. Indeed most patients are usually very concerned by their future prospects for developing dementia. It has been demonstrated that mental function is a leading factor in quality of life assessments conducted in Parkinson's disease patients and furthermore is a leading risk factor precipitating admission to nursing home care.

3.7 Prior to developing dementia, do Parkinson's disease patients have any other manifestations of disturbed thinking?

Yes, often in the form of hallucinations and confusional episodes.

In the early stages of the disease patients can often have very subtle changes in memory or thinking which can only really be detected by specialist neuropsychological tests. However, it is not uncommon in more advanced cases for the patients themselves to notice slight difficulties or problems in their ability to handle complex situations. In particular, patients often experience slight difficulty in switching from one task to another and simultaneously performing more than one activity. In many patients this level of cognitive impairment remains relatively static and may never cause overt difficulties in activities of daily living.

3.8 What are 'executive functions' and how are they impaired in Parkinson's disease?

Functions carried out in the frontal lobe, involving planning and problem solving.

Executive functions are higher-order mental tasks that demand a more complex degree of mental processing than simply remembering things. Examples of executive functions are 'working memory' and 'planning', both processes that we all use to perform mental tasks that require the holding of information in our mind and subsequently manipulating the information to achieve a solution. For example, remembering a local phone number whilst looking up an area code, then dialling the whole number together involves working memory. Likewise, planning how best to reorganise a room full of furniture without actually moving anything is another executive function. Such deficits in executive functions have clearly been demonstrated to be impaired in Parkinson's disease, even in the early stages, although this rarely affects activities of daily living.

3.9   Is there any explanation for impairment in executive functions in Parkinson's disease?

Yes, it probably relates to pathology in the frontal lobe and connections to the striatum.

It is commonly believed that executive functions are carried out in the frontal lobe cortex, whereas the major pathology in Parkinson's disease involves subcortical regions which have connections to this part of the brain. Thus it is felt that cognitive impairment in PD is primarily due to the disturbance of these circuits.

Pathological studies have, however, also shown the presence of Lewy bodies throughout the frontal cortex in PD, and it may be that the disease is affecting this cortical area directly and it is this that is responsible for the defects detected. Furthermore, cognitive impairment may also be due to pathology at other subcortical sites including the substantia nigra, the locus ceruleus, and the nucleus basalis of Meynert.

3.10   What are the causes of acute confusional state in Parkinson's disease?

Multiple causes – see Table 3.2.

Acute confusional states are common in the elderly population and even more so in patients suffering with Parkinson's disease. The causes of acute confusion in PD are essentially the same as in other elderly populations. Sudden changes in a patient's cognitive state are usually due to organic causes such as infections, or alterations in prescribed medications, and these can be reversed if recognised and treated appropriately. Another common cause for such periods of confusion is a change in environment or poor lighting after dark. As such, familiar well-lit settings and, where possible, the stabilising presence of close relatives prove to be a simple and effective measure in reducing this problem. A specific algorithm for the treatment of acute confusion in PD is given in Chapter 6 (*see* Q. 6.9).

TABLE 3.2 Causes of acute confusion in PD

Causes of acute confusion	Examples
Peripheral infection	Urinary tract infection Aspiration pneumonia secondary to impaired swallowing Infected pressure sores following prolonged poor mobility
Intracerebral pathology	Subdural haematoma with or without history of falls or head injury Encephalitis, meningitis, stroke
Medication	New anti-parkinsonian prescription Altered dose of Parkinson's disease prescription Deliberate or accidental drug overdosage
Metabolic	Poor swallowing leading to dehydration Constipation Electrolyte imbalance

3.11 Is mood affected in Parkinson's disease?

Yes, in about 40% of patients – typically depression.

About 40% of patients with Parkinson's disease normally experience a degree of depression at the time of diagnosis or during the course of the disease. Depression commonly occurs following diagnosis, and in some cases is no more than a natural reaction to this and is both transient and often mild. As the disease progresses, further patients may experience a reactive depression to new symptoms or disabilities. Only about 1–2% of patients will ever go on to develop a serious depressive condition requiring drug therapy.

3.12 Most patients with Parkinson's disease look depressed. Why is this?

This is due to facial hypomimia.

The reason why most patients with Parkinson's disease look depressed is because the slowness of movement which characterises this condition also affects the facial muscles. They often therefore have a lack of facial expressions, so-called *hypomimia*. It is therefore extremely easy to think that patients with Parkinson's disease are depressed when they are simply manifesting their disease. Many patients are unaware of this alteration in their appearance, and may be shocked when they see recent photographs of themselves. Loss of motivation or initiative are also common symptoms of PD and can add to the appearance that the patient is depressed.

3.13 What are the manifestations of mood disturbances in Parkinson's disease?

As for the condition in other situations.

There is nothing special in the mood disturbances that are seen in Parkinson's disease compared to general psychiatry. The features of depression are therefore:

- loss of appetite
- loss of sexual libido
- early morning wakening
- low self-esteem
- social withdrawal
- suicidal ideation.

In the case of mania which can be precipitated by drug therapy the features are:

- grandiose ideas
- delusional thoughts
- disjointed thinking
- overspending of money
- inappropriate and often disinhibited behaviour.

The vast majority of patients do not experience mood disturbances to this extent.

3.14 What is the best way of assessing depression in Parkinson's disease?

Using one of the standard well-validated assessments.

It is possible to be more objective in the assessment of depressive states by using tools such as the Beck Depression Inventory, the Hamilton Depression Inventory, or Geriatric Depression Scale. Patients can complete these assessments themselves between consultations, and thus provide a useful indication of whether they have significant depression, which might warrant treatment. The Geriatric Depression Scale is reproduced in Appendix 1.

3.15 Is there an underlying pathology causing depression in Parkinson's disease?

Not known, but possibly relates to a loss of brain serotonin (5-HT) activity.

Neural pathways in the brain utilising dopamine and serotonin as neurotransmitters are known to be intimately associated. Current theories of the pathophysiology in depression are related to disturbance in the serotonergic neurotransmitter pathways originating from the brainstem, so the selective serotonin reuptake inhibitor (SSRI) drugs have proved very effective in its treatment.

3.16 How common are hallucinations and psychosis in Parkinson's disease?

Relatively common and usually benign, although they can be disruptive and disturbing.

Studies of hallucinations or psychosis in Parkinson's disease have reported prevalence rates between 5–50% with visual hallucinations and paranoid delusions being the most frequent symptoms. However, the majority of these studies find that only about 20% of patients are ever affected with these types of behavioural disturbance. Hallucinations in the *early* stages of the disease, often provoked by drug therapy, should suggest the possibility of the diagnosis of dementia with Lewy bodies (*see Q. 3.3*).

3.17 What causes hallucinations and psychosis in Parkinson's disease?

Possible dopaminergic stimulation of a diseased cortex with multiple Lewy bodies.

It is widely believed that this pattern of behavioural disturbance in Parkinson's disease is the result of dopaminergic hypersensitivity and chronic exposure to dopaminergic drugs in the context of cortical pathological changes. In a system depleted of dopamine, it is known that postsynaptic receptors are upregulated in terms of both number and sensitivity and that stimulation by dopaminergic drugs could cause overactivity in these dopamine systems, leading to hallucinations and psychosis. The dopaminergic pathways most involved are those that link the midbrain dopamine neurons to the limbic and frontal cortices.

Various other factors are associated with increased frequency of hallucinations and these are listed in Box 3.2.

BOX 3.2 Factors associated with increased frequency of hallucinations

■ Greater age
■ Longer duration of illness
■ Cognitive impairment
■ Depression
■ Sleep disturbance
■ Poor visual acuity

3.18 Does the concentration of L-dopa cause hallucinations?

 No.

> Parkinson's patients known to suffer with frequent hallucinations
> have been investigated with administration of L-dopa intravenously.
> Neither a continuous infusion of high-dose L-dopa nor several pulses
> of high-dose L-dopa resulted in any change in the frequency of
> hallucinations. Thus it seems that hallucinations are not simply
> related to the concentration of L-dopa or to sudden fluctuations in
> its levels, but nevertheless they do seem to have some relationship
> to dopaminergic therapies.

3.19 Are there any specific features of hallucinations in Parkinson's disease?

Yes – typically visual.

Hallucinations in Parkinson's disease are typically visual in nature (although auditory and tactile episodes have been reported), are usually non-threatening, and occur more frequently at night, while the patient is alert with the eyes open. Most commonly, the affected individual sees blurred images of people (often deceased family members) or animals, lasting for seconds or minutes. Insight is usually preserved and the patient is aware that the hallucinations are not real. However, in some cases they can be frightening, fuelling and promoting paranoid delusions.

3.20 What are the major problems caused by hallucinations and psychosis in Parkinson's disease?

Disturbed behaviour and a tendency to earlier nursing home placement.

In addition to the obvious distress caused to both patients and family, this aspect of Parkinson's disease has significant implications. Hallucinations have been demonstrated to be a strong risk factor for admission to nursing homes. One study comparing PD patients admitted to nursing home care with patients able to remain in their own homes revealed no difference between physical disability and mental impairment, but a significant difference in the presence and severity of hallucinations. Furthermore, of those admitted to nursing homes, none returned home and all died within 2 years.

PQ PATIENT QUESTIONS

Am I going to lose my marbles?

There is no reason to think that you are going to lose your memory or ability to think. Parkinson's disease is predominantly a disorder that impairs movements, and impairment of memory does not necessarily occur and is by no means inevitable. Even if you feel that your memory is worse than it used to be already, you may notice improved memory and that you can think more clearly after we start you on anti-Parkinson's treatment. These drugs can increase your alertness and concentration, and also improve your speech, which may help you join in conversations more fully and enjoy social interactions more.

My partner thinks I'm depressed, but wouldn't you be?

People with Parkinson's disease often look depressed to other people even when they are not. This is because the muscles of the face are affected by the disease and become slower in showing expressions and emotions. This might be what your partner has noticed. It is also not uncommon for patients to describe a loss of interest in doing new things, and again this can be misinterpreted as depression. Treatment of your Parkinson's disease may help all of these features. It is possible, however, that you will have periods of feeling genuinely depressed in response to your symptoms, but fortunately these 'low' periods tend to be temporary for most Parkinson's patients. If you feel depressed for a sustained period, it may be necessary to consider tablets specifically for depression.

Confirming the diagnosis of Parkinson's disease

4

4.1 Can the diagnosis of Parkinson's disease be confirmed in life?

No.

> There are no tests in life to confirm that someone has Parkinson's disease, outside of those very few centres which have specialised PET scanners and even then it is hard to be absolutely certain (*see Q. 4.6*). The diagnosis of Parkinson's disease therefore relies on the experience of the doctor seeing the patient, recognising the early symptoms of the diseases and fully assessing the patient's clinical features (*see Q. 1.25*).

4.2 How can one be certain that a patient has Parkinson's disease?

One cannot, the only definite way is at post-mortem.

Clinicopathological studies suggest that up to 20–30% of patients diagnosed with Parkinson's disease during life have alternative causes for their symptoms when the brain is examined after death (*see Q. 1.25*). This high rate of misdiagnosis can be minimised by referral of patients for specialist opinion, and regular review of the evolution of the disease and its response to treatment with anti-parkinsonian drugs.

4.3 When should I refer Parkinson's disease patients to specialist clinics?

Early on in the presentation (*Fig. 4.1*).

There are now many physicians running specialist Parkinson's disease clinics within the UK. At the onset of disease, the diagnosis can be difficult to make with certainty and may be confused with normal ageing, the stiffness of arthritis, the cognitive slowing of Alzheimer's disease or benign forms of tremor. Early specialist opinions can both facilitate diagnosis, and coordinate initiation of drug therapy. Specialist clinics can also provide the early involvement of PD nurses, physiotherapists, occupational therapists and support groups. Most specialists would request that patients are referred as soon as they present with any symptoms suspicious of PD, prior to the institution of any anti-PD treatment. This is so that the signs of the disease may be assessed without the possibility of diagnostic confusion that sometimes occurs in patients already started on anti-PD treatment, although an excellent response to therapy may help in establishing the diagnosis.

At a patient's first visit, discussion of the diagnosis should include addressing the common misconceptions lay people have about the diagnosis of PD. As PD progresses, patients can suffer from increased passivity and lack of motivation and an active treatment programme early

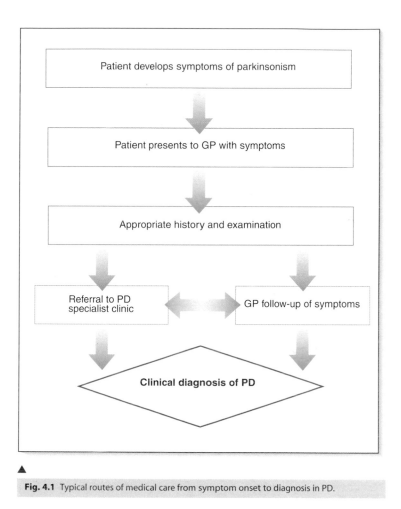

Fig. 4.1 Typical routes of medical care from symptom onset to diagnosis in PD.

in the disease can avoid this. Unfortunately, not all regions of the UK have access to specialist PD clinics, and it then becomes even more important for the GP to coordinate the multidisciplinary approach to patient management.

4.4   Should I refer patients to a neurologist or a geriatrician?

Probably best in the first instance to send them to a local Parkinson's disease expert, irrespective of the expert's specialty.

Parkinson's disease is a not-infrequent cause for referral to both geriatrician- and neurologist-led outpatient clinics, and within either medical discipline, individual doctors frequently sub-specialise in particular diseases including PD. When a region is fortunate enough to have a recognised specialist with a particular interest in PD, clearly he or she will be the most up-to-date source of advice for patients of any age. In regions without identified PD specialists, the decision on who to refer to should be based on a combination of age and the presence of co-morbidity.

The majority of patients with suspected PD are between 50 and 80 years of age at the onset of their disease. Patients who are both 'chronologically' and 'biologically' young and have active lifestyles would not expect to be referred to a geriatrician for assessment of their symptoms, and will be best followed up in a neurology clinic. Patients who are more dependent and may require assistance at home, or consideration of alternative accommodation, may be better assessed within a geriatric clinic setting.

4.5 How does brain imaging help in Parkinson's disease?

It is normally helpful in excluding other causes of parkinsonism.

The scans which most people have for Parkinson's disease are either CT (computerised tomography) or MRI (magnetic resonance imaging) scans of the brain. Both types of scan reveal the structure of the brain, but both are typically normal in PD because the problem relates to a loss of a small group of nerve cells releasing dopamine, which is too small to be detectable on structural imaging. Occasionally patients will have slightly abnormal scans, in which case the possibility of secondary parkinsonism is raised, as opposed to idiopathic Parkinson's disease (*see Ch. 10*). In these cases, the parkinsonian features relate to either strokes or some other structural lesion, damaging the basal ganglia regions of the brain. A sudden onset of symptoms, headaches, or the presence of non-parkinsonian neurological signs (e.g. spasticity or sensory loss) may suggest a vascular aetiology or structural lesion, and these patients should certainly be investigated with brain imaging. Patients who have typical features of PD, occurring after middle age, almost always have normal brain scans, and many clinicians feel that there is little information to be gained by performing these investigations. However, if there is any doubt, or anxiety that the patient has anything other than PD, then a scan should be performed; indeed many patients feel unhappy at not having such an investigation (see Patient questions at the end of this chapter).

4.6   What is positron-emission tomography or PET scanning?

A special type of scan that detects chemicals within the brain, available in one or two specialist research centres in the UK – not of use to patients attending normal clinics.

Positron-emission tomography (PET) scanning is a procedure in which chemicals can be visualised within the brain. The procedure involves the intravenous injection of a small amount of a radioactive compound, which is subsequently taken up by specific areas of the brain. In the case of Parkinson's disease the chemical that has been commonly used is a substance called fluoro-dopa, which is taken up by the remaining dopamine cells within the brain. Where there is a loss of these dopamine cells and dopamine terminals in the striatum, there is a loss of chemical uptake, and therefore lower levels of fluoro-dopa are seen in the striatum (*Fig. 4.2*).

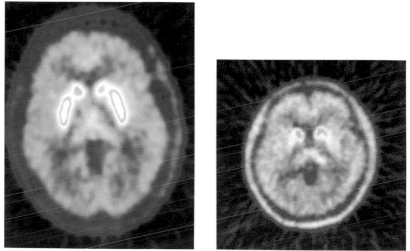

▲
Fig. 4.2 Appearance of fluoro-dopa PET scans: **A.** normal; **B.** PD patient. Courtesy of Dr Paola Piccini, Hammersmith Hospital, London.

Many parkinsonian conditions have deficiencies of fluoro-dopa in the striatum, but it is the pattern of loss that is often helpful in diagnosing Parkinson's disease, and making distinctions from Parkinson-plus syndromes (*see Ch. 10*). In the latter conditions, striatal uptake of fluoro-dopa dopaminergic markers tends to be equally decreased in both the putamen and caudate parts of the striatum, in contrast to the preferential involvement of the posterior putamen in PD.

PET scanning exists in only a few specialist centres as there is a need to:

- make the radioactive substances nearby, since these substances decay very rapidly, and
- access very sophisticated computing machinery and expertise that is required for image acquisition and analysis.

As a result there are very few centres around the UK that can perform PET scans and as such they are reserved and used for research purposes. Therefore patients sent to clinics will not be scanned using PET unless recruited to specific research projects.

4.7 What is a DaTSCAN?

A more available, but less sensitive nuclear medicine scan, used to detect dopamine activity in the striatum.

Another type of functional scan that has been developed for use in PD uses SPECT (single photon emission computerised tomography) technology, and a radioligand – [^{123}I]-FP-CIT, which is also taken up in the striatum of normal brains (*Fig. 4.3*). For ease of reference these scans are commercially referred to as DaTSCANs. The resolution that these scans produce is not as high as that seen in PET scanning but the equipment is more widely available in nuclear medicine departments. Recent studies have confirmed high levels of sensitivity and specificity in the differentiation of individuals with parkinsonism from those with essential tremor.

These scans, because they are more readily available than PET scans, may have some use in certain individuals where the clinical diagnosis is in doubt, although their diagnostic power has yet to be fully determined.

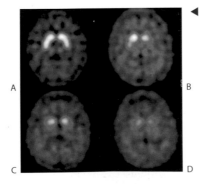

Fig. 4.3 Appearance of normal and PD brains using DaTSCAN: **A.** healthy control; **B.** patient with Parkinson's disease (Hoehn and Yahr stage 1 – *see Box 1.2*); **C.** patient with essential tremor; **D.** patient with advanced stage PD (Hoehn and Yahr stage 4). Reproduced with permission of Amersham Health (www.amershamhealth.com, www.datscan.com).

4.8   Are these types of brain scan safe?

Yes, but the number any individual can have is limited when radioisotopes are employed.

Straightforward CT scans are routine investigations and whilst they require a patient to be exposed to radiation to produce detailed images, the levels are considered acceptably safe. MRI scans are completely free from harmful radiation, although occasional allergic reactions can be seen when contrast agents are given in both MRI (gadolinium) and CT.

PET and SPECT scans require the injection of radioactive isotopes and whilst these are not considered harmful to human tissues, it restricts the number of scans any individual patient can have. Furthermore, PET and SPECT scans do require patients to be free from dopaminergic therapies, and even temporary cessation of treatments may be associated with increased morbidity.

4.9   What is an L-dopa challenge?

A way of assessing response to treatment using a single-dose oral L-dopa challenge.

A good symptomatic response to L-dopa has been shown to increase the likelihood of a correct diagnosis of Parkinson's disease. As a result, some clinicians have tried using single doses of L-dopa as a 'challenge' to assess a patient's response. Unfortunately many genuine PD patients with mild symptoms early on in the disease do not notice any beneficial response to single doses of L-dopa, and some patients with atypical parkinsonian syndromes may sense some benefit from such a single dose. As such, the results of L-dopa challenge tests can be hard to interpret. Furthermore, there is evidence that even a single dose of L-dopa may increase the risk of the subsequent development of dyskinesias above that seen following dopamine agonist treatment (see Q. 5.9). If the decision to start treatment with L-dopa has been taken, it is more diagnostically informative to continue the treatment trial with adequate doses for some months before concluding that L-dopa therapy is ineffective. In these circumstances the likelihood of diagnoses other than PD is significantly higher.

4.10   What is an apomorphine test?

An alternative approach to testing the dopaminergic responsiveness of patients and thus the likelihood that they have Parkinson's disease.

An apomorphine test is another 'challenge test' (Box 4.1) that has been devised to see whether a patient will respond to standard dopamine therapy for Parkinson's disease. (Apomorphine as a treatment for PD is discussed separately (see Qs 7.17–7.20).) Although the sensitivity and specificity of this test is again questionable, there is no increased risk of dyskinesias following

---

BOX 4.1 The apomorphine test

- Patient suspected of having Parkinson's disease
- All anti-PD treatments are stopped
- Patient pretreated with oral domperidone 20 mg t.d.s. for 3–4 days
- Arrangement for admission to hospital
- Patient symptoms assessed objectively, e.g. number of finger taps in 30 seconds
- Patient given successively increasing doses of subcutaneous apomorphine:
  - 1 mg
  - 2 mg
  - 3 mg
  - 5 mg
- Patient re-assessed 15 minutes after each dose until there is objective improvement or the patient feels unwell

---

this type of test and therefore it is unlikely to be of any harm to the patient. The test is best done in hospital, and accurate measures of response assessment need to be made. Patients must be treated with adequate doses of the antiemetic domperidone before the trial, otherwise the patient will vomit. Domperidone *has* to be used rather than other standard antiemetics (such as metoclopramide or prochlorperazine) because it does not cross the blood–brain barrier and bind to dopamine receptors in the brain.

4.11 Are any other tests necessary in patients suspected of having Parkinson's disease?

Only if you suspect that the patient may have secondary parkinsonism. This is usually in atypical cases.

It should be emphasised to all patients with parkinsonism that there are no diagnostic tests to *confirm* the diagnosis of Parkinson's disease or the Parkinson-plus disorders. Despite this, some patients should be given simple blood tests to *exclude* a variety of possible causes for their symptoms (*Table 4.1*). Blood tests are of limited value in the investigation of patients with typical PD, although any patients with tremor certainly should have simple thyroid function tests performed. Concurrent liver disease or the presence of Kayser–Fleischer rings on the iris should rouse the suspicion of Wilson's disease, which can be screened for by testing serum copper and caeruloplasmin levels, and urine copper levels. *This should be performed in all patients with onset of PD below 40 years* since complete resolution of symptoms together with a normal life span can follow accurate diagnosis and treatment of patients with Wilson's disease (see Q. 10.12).

Lumbar puncture and CSF examination has been used in the past to measure the levels of metabolites of dopamine but these tests are not a reliable indicator of the disease and are therefore now no longer performed.

TABLE 4.1 Investigations that should be performed in patients with parkinsonism

Investigation	Contributory information
Full blood count (FBC)	Presence of anaemia contributing to lethargy, dizziness or slowing down
Erythrocyte sedimentation rate (ESR)	Suspicion of occult malignancy, vasculitis or infection causing focal neurological signs or lethargy
Thyroid function	Hyperthyroidism causing tremor Hypothyroidism causing lethargy
Vitamin B_{12}	Unsteadiness or gait difficulty due to peripheral neuropathy and/or subacute combined degeneration of the cord
Copper and caeruloplasmin	Undiagnosed Wilson's disease causing young-onset parkinsonism
CT or MRI brain imaging*	Rule out a space-occupying lesion, hydrocephalus or vascular lesions

* Imaging tests usually only provide useful information if there are atypical features of the disease (see Qs 4.5 and 4.8).

4.12 What are the Parkinson-plus syndromes?

Rare conditions in which there is degeneration of several systems in the brain leading to parkinsonism as well as other major neurological problems.

Parkinson-plus syndromes consist of a series of conditions in which the pathology extends out of the nigrostriatal system and involves either the autonomic nervous system, the balance centre at the back of the brain (cerebellum) or the cortex and its descending motor pathways. Characteristically these disorders run a more rapidly progressive course than idiopathic Parkinson's disease and respond less well to therapy. The Parkinson-plus syndromes are discussed in Chapter 10.

4.13 **What are the main points I should emphasise to a patient, once the diagnosis of Parkinson's disease has been made?**

See Box 4.2.

BOX 4.2 Points to discuss with a patient initially diagnosed with Parkinson's disease

- The nature and natural history of Parkinson's disease
- The types of treatment and expected response
- Lack of familial risk for the majority of Parkinson's disease
- Other sources of support that may help
- The role of the hospital

It is often extremely difficult in the early stages to be certain of the diagnosis of Parkinson's disease, and both the doctor and patient can find this frustrating. It is also true to say that patients often fail to take in much information when the initial diagnosis is passed on to them. The important points that the patient needs to grasp are:

1. PD is incurable and runs a progressive course over a decade or two. The symptoms occur because of a loss of certain brain cells within the brainstem.

2. The treatment is palliative not curative, but there are many therapies which are extremely helpful, especially in the early stages. Furthermore, much research is being done to improve these drug therapies along with strategies for helping the patient in the later stages of the disease.

3. There is no evidence that the disease is inherited for the vast majority of patients, so that they do not need to worry about other family members, unless a strong family history is elicited during the consultation.

4. There are support organisations for people with PD, in particular the Parkinson's Disease Society, which is both a national organisation and has local branches. This is a useful way of meeting other people with similar symptoms, and keeping up-to-date with breakthroughs and research (*see Q. 11.5*). Attendance at meetings is not essential for these updates as the society also produces a regular newsletter.

5. Treatments for PD can often be extremely complicated, and regular medical or neurological review of patient therapies is advisable.

PQ PATIENT QUESTIONS

Shouldn't I have a brain scan?

There is normally no need for you to have a brain scan. Many patients share your feeling that there should be a definitive test to tell them whether they have Parkinson's disease before they can be sure that the diagnosis is correct. Unfortunately there is no such test available. Sometimes we arrange CT or MRI scans which look at the structure of the brain to exclude other possible conditions in patients with symptoms that are not completely typical of Parkinson's disease. In fact, a number of people actually find brain scans quite uncomfortable and claustrophobic, and whilst the risks associated with brain scans are small, it is not necessary to have such a procedure unless we are concerned that there is something else causing the parkinsonism. By far the most likely explanation for your symptoms is Parkinson's disease; however, there will always be a degree of 'uncertainty' surrounding the diagnosis, and whilst this uncertainty changes with time and responses to therapy, we can only be completely certain of the diagnosis at post-mortem.

Can't you test my blood for Parkinson's disease?

Unfortunately no. There is no blood test that can confirm the presence of Parkinson's disease. Occasionally, we do blood tests to ensure that you are free from other diseases that share similar symptoms to Parkinson's, or can occur at the same time as Parkinson's, but there is no laboratory that can give us a yes or no answer. However, as genetic causes for Parkinson's disease are being recognised in certain families and young patients, then some genetic blood tests may in the future become more routine.

Are you sure I have Parkinson's disease?

It is impossible to be 100% sure that any patient has Parkinson's disease, although it is far more common than any of the other conditions that have similar symptoms. As the years pass, we can become *more certain* that you have Parkinson's rather than any of the more rare forms of 'parkinsonism', since the other forms of parkinsonism tend not to respond to treatment, and other symptoms quite distinct from those of Parkinson's disease develop. If you have any problems with falls, problems with reading, dizzy spells or urinary system problems, then we will arrange some further tests to find out if you have one of the more unusual 'Parkinson syndromes'.

The priority is to treat your disease with drugs when they are required, and monitor any benefit that they give you. It will also be necessary to check on other ways to make sure that your symptoms are neither too much of a nuisance or a hazard for you.

Drug treatment of early Parkinson's disease (motor symptoms) **5**

5.1   When should treatment be started for a patient with Parkinson's disease?

As soon as symptoms start to interfere significantly with employment or activities of daily living.

There is a temptation once the diagnosis has been made to immediately start a patient on treatment for Parkinson's disease. However, it is sensible to wait until treatment is indicated, and this is normally at a point when the symptoms are significantly interfering with activities of daily living or employment. Obviously this varies from patient to patient and job to job. For example when tremor is dominant, and the patient is a fine craftsman, then treatment will need to be started earlier than in a bradykinetic rigid patient in whom slowed speed of movement is not having any impact on lifestyle. Patients should be involved in the decision-making process throughout and they should be provided with sufficient information about PD and the rationale for drug treatment to allow them to make an informed decision about when they would like to start receiving treatment.

Non-drug therapies should also be considered at the onset of the disease. Patients are best able to learn new strategies while their motor and cognitive functions are relatively preserved, and so referral to the services of occupational therapists and physiotherapists should not be delayed until the disease is advanced (see Ch. 9). When available, these services are best sought through a specialist PD clinic. Finally, early involvement of the PD specialist nurse is advised, and this can help with decisions on drug and non-drug therapies at this stage of the illness.

5.2   Are there guidelines for the treatment of Parkinson's disease?

Yes, but treatment still needs to be decided on an individual basis.

Guidelines for the management of Parkinson's disease are produced on a regular basis, following consensus meetings by various panels of specialists, expert in the treatment of PD. The response of an individual patient to any of the drug preparations is not always predictable and therefore guidelines should be used as an aid to therapy rather than being followed obsessively. A sensible guide for the treatment of PD patients is shown in Figure 5.1. Failure or intolerance of one particular drug may require substitution of another drug of the same class prior to proceeding to a drug of another class.

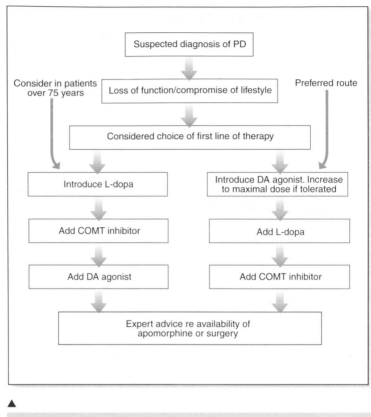

▲

Fig. 5.1 Guidelines for the treatment of Parkinson's disease.

5.3   Who should start treatment for the Parkinson's disease patient?

If in doubt, await decision of specialist for initiation of therapy.

Most specialists would prefer to see patients before they are started on treatment in order to fully assess the extent of their symptoms, and then make a recommendation on appropriate treatment. Where referral to such a specialist clinic is possible within a reasonable time period, treatment ought to be withheld pending this assessment, and this decision discussed with the patient. In some regions, early specialist opinions are not available and the decision regarding the choice and the timing of drug therapy rests with patients and their GP.

5.4   What drug should be started first?

 Probably a dopamine agonist, but it depends on the age and dominant symptom at presentation.

It is still unresolved as to which treatment is best in the early stages of Parkinson's disease. Certainly the gold standard of treatment is L-dopa (Sinemet or Madopar). However, there is increasing evidence that dopamine agonists are almost as effective as L-dopa in the early stages of the disease and also have the benefit that they delay some of the long-term motor complications that are seen with L-dopa, most notably dyskinesias (*see Q. 7.11*).

Elderly patients are less likely to need anti-PD therapy for so long a time, and therefore they run a lower risk of suffering from the long-term complications of L-dopa therapy. In addition, elderly patients suffer more morbidity from the short-term side-effects of hallucinations, somnolence and freezing which occur more commonly with the dopamine agonists. It is therefore sensible to consider using L-dopa as the first-line treatment in these patients. Younger patients who are in desperate need of rapid and complete resolution of symptoms should be given a full and frank discussion of the risks and benefits of L-dopa and the dopamine agonist drugs, and encouraged to be involved in the decision regarding which drug to start first. Where employment is in jeopardy, L-dopa is more likely to restore function more rapidly. Generally, however, patients below the age of 65, or above the age of 65 with no other co-morbidity are started on a dopamine agonist as initial monotherapy.

5.5   Will drug treatment reverse all of the Parkinson's disease symptoms?

Possibly, although tremor and gait problems respond less well to dopaminergic therapy.

All the features of Parkinson's disease respond to dopaminergic drug treatment in the early stages of the disease, although tremor and walking abnormalities often respond least well. Where tremor is the most disabling feature of the disease, consideration should be given to the use of anticholinergic therapies or β-blockers (*see Qs 5.28 and 5.29*). With time, all treatments become less effective and a number of other problems related to the disease or its treatment may arise which might require special treatment (*see Ch. 7*).

5.6   What is a dopamine agonist?

A drug that directly binds and activates dopamine receptors in the brain and by so doing mimics the effects of dopamine.

There are now many chemicals which have been synthesised that bind to one or several of the receptors for dopamine in the brain. Such drugs on binding stimulate the receptor, in contrast to antagonists which bind to the receptors and prevent the normal chemical from acting. So-called 'partial agonists' cause some stimulation of the receptor but less than that produced by the natural transmitter dopamine, and thus partially diminish the response of the cell to endogenous dopamine release. Indeed some drugs can be an agonist to one type of receptor and antagonistic to other types of dopamine receptor (e.g. bromocriptine). In general, dopamine agonists activate dopamine receptors and thus mimic the effects of dopamine in the brain

5.7 What dopamine agonists are available?

A variety of such drugs exist, with ropinirole and cabergoline being the most favoured at the present time.

Dopamine agonists have been used in Parkinson's disease for many years. There are a range of drugs that form this class of compounds (*Table 5.1*), of which the earliest agents were bromocriptine and lisuride. These have now been superseded by drugs with slightly better side-effect profiles and longer half-lives making them more effective for longer periods of time. Of course there are still patients who have been successfully treated

TABLE 5.1 The range of dopamine agonists

Drug	Structure	Actions	Cautions
Bromocriptine	Ergot	D_2 agonist, D_1 antagonist	Hypotensive reactions
Lisuride	Ergot	D_2 agonist, D_1 antagonist	Severe peripheral vascular disease, coronary disease
Pergolide	Ergot	D_1 and D_2 agonist	History of cardiac disease, or confusion
Ropinirole	Non-ergot	D_2 agonist	Cardiac disease, major psychoses, hepatic and renal impairment
Cabergoline	Ergot	D_2 agonist	Hypotensive reactions
Pramipexole	Non-ergot	D_2 and D_3 agonist	Renal impairment, psychoses
Apomorphine	Non-ergot	D_1 and D_2 agonist	Postural hypotension, cognitive impairment

with the older dopamine agonists for many years and such patients should remain on these drugs if their symptoms are well controlled. Change for the sake of it is not recommended. The newer dopamine agonists, cabergoline, ropinirole, and pramipexole, are generally better tolerated by PD patients and these should tend to be used for newly diagnosed patients.

In addition, there is an injectable dopamine agonist called apomorphine. This drug has absolutely no similarity whatsoever to morphine and activates dopamine receptors. Apomorphine is especially effective for patients who have difficulty swallowing tablets, as it is injectable subcutaneously, and/or in patients who have severe 'off' periods (*see* Q. 7.17), as it can act rapidly in the brain and by so doing converts the 'off' period into 'on' time. It can also be used as a continuous infusion in advanced PD (*see* Q. 7.20).

5.8   How should a dopamine agonist be started?

 At low dose, then increasing towards the maximum dose dictated by clinical benefits or side-effects.

Dopamine agonists work by directly binding to dopamine receptors and therefore mimic what dopamine does normally in the brain. Unfortunately many of these drugs also bind at sites outside of the striatum, including the vomiting centre in the brainstem. Some patients therefore require an additional antiemetic such as domperidone (a dopamine antagonist), which does not cross the blood–brain barrier, but blocks the emetic affects of these dopamine agonists. Dopamine agonists should be started in low doses and increased gradually over a series of weeks. If the drug is increased too rapidly, patients are likely to feel very unwell and stop the medication themselves. The scheme for starting any of the modern dopamine agonists is represented in Table 5.2. Fortunately, several of these drugs are produced in 'starter packs', which greatly simplifies the dose increments for patients.

5.9   What are the side-effects of the dopamine agonists?

Nausea, vomiting, postural hypotension and confusion with hallucinations.

All side-effects can be minimised through the slow and gradual introduction of these drugs. However, constipation, fatigue, nausea, postural hypotension and vivid dreams do regularly occur, as well as multiple infrequently reported side-effects. Although less common than with L-dopa, dyskinesias and painful dystonic spasms may also occur with prolonged use. Hallucinations may be experienced by up to a quarter of patients treated with the ergot forms of dopamine agonist, although these are often brief and not too distressing to the patient. Reduction in medication may, however, be necessary for the relief of these symptoms which can be more distressing for the family and carer than the patient. If dopamine agonists are to be withdrawn, then the drugs should be slowly reduced.

TABLE 5.2 Initiation of dopamine agonist treatment

Drug	Starting dose	Initial dose increments	Later dose increments	Target dose
Pergolide	50 μg o.d.	Increase by 100 μg every third day. Give in 3 divided doses	After day 12, increase by 250 μg every third day	1 mg t.d.s.
Ropinirole	250 μg t.d.s.	Increase by 250 μg t.d.s. at weekly intervals	Above 1 mg t.d.s., may increase by a further 1 mg t.d.s. at weekly intervals	6–8 mg t.d.s.
Cabergoline	1 mg o.d.	Increase by 1 mg daily at weekly intervals		2–6 mg o.d.
Pramipexole	125 μg t.d.s.	Increase by 125 μg t.d.s. at weekly intervals	Increase by 250 μg t.d.s. at weekly intervals	1.5 mg t.d.s.

Abrupt cessation of dopamine agonists theoretically may precipitate a *neuroleptic-type malignant syndrome*, characterised by hyperthermia, confusion, rigidity and autonomic dysequilibrium. If this occurs, urgent referral is required to a local medical team with access to an intensive care unit.

5.10 Do dopamine agonists cause sleep attacks?

Yes in some rare cases.

Several reports of sudden sleep attacks occurring in PD patients while driving roused concern that the dopamine agonists caused sleep attacks. Initially, ropinirole was thought to be the most culpable, but further studies have shown excessive daytime sleepiness to be associated with all of the dopamine agonists and L-dopa. The Epworth sleepiness scale (*see Fig. 2.1*) can be used to assess sleepiness in PD patients, following which patients should be educated about the soporific effects of both PD and the medications used to treat it, and if they suffer from persistent daytime sleepiness they should be advised against driving.

5.11 What are the important drug interactions of the dopamine agonists?

Primarily with drugs that block dopamine receptors such as major tranquillisers and antiemetics.

Most of the known drug interactions of the dopamine agonists apply to all members of the group equally. Obviously, dopamine antagonist antiemetics such as metoclopramide or prochlorperazine reduce the effectiveness of the dopamine agonists and should not be used. Domperidone does not cross the blood–brain barrier and is the preferred antiemetic in all cases of PD. Antipsychotic drugs also reduce the anti-parkinsonian effect of these drugs through dopamine antagonism. Erythromycin and sympathomimetic drugs can increase the plasma levels of the dopamine agonists, and can potentially lead to toxicity. Cimetidine can also inhibit the excretion of pramipexole.

5.12 What are the relative costs of the dopamine agonists?

See Table 5.3.

5.13 What is L-dopa and how does it work?

The precursor of dopamine, which works by being taken up in the brain by the remaining dopamine nerve cells and converted into dopamine, which is then released.

L-dopa is the precursor to the neurotransmitter dopamine, which is released by the nigral neurons in the striatum. Unfortunately, one cannot give dopamine to a patient orally as it has major effects on blood pressure, is largely broken down in the body and does not cross the blood–brain barrier. L-dopa, on the other hand, is taken up through the gut, then into the brain and finally into the surviving nerve terminals, where it is converted into the active compound dopamine. L-dopa therapy therefore requires a number of intact presynaptic dopaminergic neurons so that it can be metabolised to dopamine, in order to have an effect. Excess dopamine may then be released from these surviving nerve terminals to compensate for the dopamine deficiency state caused by Parkinson's disease (see Fig. 1.1).

5.14 Is levodopa the same as L-dopa?

Yes.

L-dopa is an abbreviation of levodopa, which is metabolised to the active transmitter dopamine after being taken up into the surviving nerve terminals.

Drug	Manufacturer (Trade name)	Maintenance dose range	Typical daily dose	Annual cost of typical daily dose
Bromocriptine	Novartis (Parlodel)	10–40 mg	20 mg	£463.77
Lisuride	Non-proprietary	0.6–5 mg	1.2 mg	£918.05
Pramipexole	Pharmacia (Mirapexin)	1.5–4.5 mg	1.5 mg	£1162.01
Cabergoline	Pharmacia (Cabaser)	2–6 mg	4 mg	£1376.96
Pergolide	Lilly (Celance)	1–5 mg	3 mg	£1611.29
Ropinirole	Glaxo-SmithKline (Requip)	6–18 mg	12 mg	£2409.00
Apomorphine	Britannia (Britaject)	3–100 mg	25 mg (s.c. infusion)	£2910.88

TABLE 5.3 The relative costs of the dopamine agonists

5.15 How should L-dopa be started?

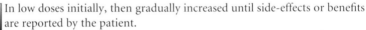

In low doses initially, then gradually increased until side-effects or benefits are reported by the patient.

All L-dopa preparations should be gradually introduced, but there is still much variation in clinician prescribing habits. 100 mg/day of L-dopa is the traditional starting dose for frail or elderly patients, which might be as Madopar 62.5 twice daily, or Sinemet 62.5 twice daily. (Both of these tablet formulations contain 50 mg of L-dopa.) The daily dose of L-dopa should be increased by 100 mg after 1 week, and by the same amount after 2 weeks. If tolerated, further increases should be reviewed after 6–12 weeks on this dose.

Less caution is required for younger or more robust patients who receive more initial benefit by starting on a higher dose, e.g. one tablet of Sinemet 110 t.d.s. or Madopar 125 t.d.s. This dose can be reviewed after 4–6 weeks, and further increases made according to response.

5.16 What is the difference between L-dopa, Sinemet and Madopar?

The addition of a dopa decarboxylase inhibitor to the preparation.

L-dopa is metabolised by the enzyme dopa decarboxylase in the periphery. Without an inhibitor of this enzyme, L-dopa must be given in enormous doses to reach the brain in sufficient quantities to have an effect on symptoms of parkinsonism. Such high doses would lead to severe side-effects of nausea and postural hypotension.

L-dopa preparations are therefore manufactured together with an

TABLE 5.4 Doses of the preparations of Sinemet and Madopar

	L-dopa (mg)	Decarboxylase inhibitor (mg)	Colour of tablets	Cost per 100 tablets
Madopar capsules				
62.5	50	12.5	Blue/grey	£6.67
125	100	25	Blue/pink	£9.29
250	200	50	Blue/caramel	£15.84
Madopar tablets – dispersible				
62.5	50	12.5	White scored	£7.92
125	100	25	White scored	£14.04
Madopar CR				
125	100	25	Dark green/ light blue	£17.06
Sinemet tablets				
62.5	50	12.5	Yellow scored	£7.81
110	100	10	Blue scored	£8.17
Plus – 25/100	100	25	Yellow scored	£12.01
275	250	25	Blue scored	£17.07
Sinemet CR				
25/100	100	25	Pink	£31.65
50/200	200	50	Peach	£37.25

inhibitor of dopa decarboxylase, known as carbidopa in Sinemet preparations and benserazide in Madopar preparations.

5.17 Why are there so many different types of Sinemet and Madopar?

To allow flexibility in the treatment of the condition.

The different forms of Sinemet and Madopar contain different amounts of the active ingredient L-dopa, as well as various amounts of the inhibitor preventing its breakdown in the periphery. The relative contribution of each dose is represented in Table 5.4. The advantage of having so many formulations is that one can titrate the dose of the medication very carefully for the patient's need. Furthermore, occasional patients seem to tolerate one preparation (Sinemet or Madopar) better than the other.

5.18 What is the difference between CR preparations and normal Sinemet or Madopar formulations?

CR preparations release L-dopa slowly over 8–12 hours, unlike the normal preparations which release it over a much shorter period of time.

The CR in the name of these preparations refers to 'controlled release'. These preparations were devised to have the advantage that the active ingredient would be released over an 8-hour period, rather than 2–4 hours, as is normal for most doses of Sinemet or Madopar. These drugs were therefore introduced as a way of trying to produce a smoother control of the Parkinson's disease during the day and especially at night when standard L-dopa preparations wear off. They are therefore used primarily to smooth out the control of Parkinson's disease and to help with nocturnal or early morning symptoms.

One can occasionally run into problems with using CR preparations, if they are the only drug being taken. The first problem that patients encounter is that the controlled-release preparation takes some time to enter the circulation in sufficient quantities. Thus, simply taking a controlled-release preparation first thing in the morning may not be sufficient and so can delay any benefit of the treatment for a number of hours. It is therefore often advised that the best way to use controlled-release preparations is together with standard Sinemet or Madopar first thing in the morning to 'kick-start' the patient. The second problem is that repeated doses of a controlled-release preparation can lead to progressive, somewhat erratic accumulations of L-dopa in the body, such that some patients experience severe problems in the evening with overdosage from L-dopa and dyskinesias.

5.19 What are the common side-effects of L-dopa?

Nausea, vomiting, postural hypotension and confusion with hallucinations in the short term. Unpredictable responses with dyskinesias in the long term.

There are a number of problems with these drugs, which are summarised in Box 5.1. The main side-effects that patients complain of are nausea and vomiting, postural hypotension (feeling faint on standing), and in some cases confusion and hallucinations.

Nausea and vomiting often occur at the onset of L-dopa therapy. This may be helped by taking the medication with a snack or by increasing the dose of the decarboxylase inhibitor in the tablets. Domperidone is a dopamine antagonist which does not cross the blood–brain barrier and can diminish nausea without worsening symptoms of PD, whereas other dopamine antagonists such as metoclopramide should be avoided. Cyclizine acts on cholinergic receptors and is another useful alternative to domperidone. Postural hypotension is also not uncommon, and can be ameliorated by simple advice about avoiding sudden postural changes (e.g. suddenly standing up), or in some cases using elastic compression stockings and medications such as fludrocortisone.

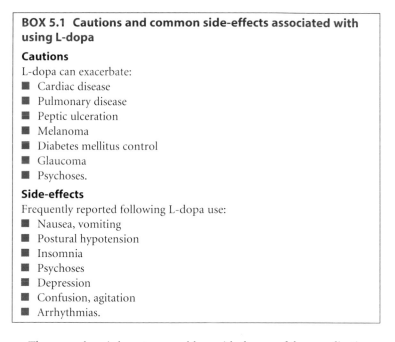

BOX 5.1 Cautions and common side-effects associated with using L-dopa

Cautions

L-dopa can exacerbate:
- Cardiac disease
- Pulmonary disease
- Peptic ulceration
- Melanoma
- Diabetes mellitus control
- Glaucoma
- Psychoses.

Side-effects

Frequently reported following L-dopa use:
- Nausea, vomiting
- Postural hypotension
- Insomnia
- Psychoses
- Depression
- Confusion, agitation
- Arrhythmias.

The more chronic long-term problem with the use of these medications is in the development of 'on/off' phenomena in which patients swing from being completely 'off' (i.e. extremely parkinsonian) to being 'on' (i.e. full of movement, often with abnormal involuntary dyskinetic movements). These symptoms often respond in the first instance to modification of the therapy, but ultimately limit the usefulness of L-dopa (*see Ch. 7*).

5.20 Should L-dopa be taken with food?

Not necessarily. It depends on how well the patient tolerates the drug.

The instructions that accompany L-dopa tablets recommend that the medication is taken with food. This is to minimise the nausea or indigestion that is experienced by the patient when L-dopa is first taken. The majority of people develop a tolerance for L-dopa over the first year of treatment such that it can usually be taken on an empty stomach. This can be of benefit to those patients who suffer weight gain due to frequent snacks taken to accompany difficult L-dopa regimes. In advanced disease, some patients notice that food diminishes the efficacy of the L-dopa because protein in the diet competes with L-dopa for uptake in the gut and brain (*see Q. 9.11*).

In general, all other anti-PD medications can be taken at any time.

5.21 Are there any important drug interactions involving L-dopa?

Yes, especially involving antihypertensives and major tranquillisers.

In addition to causing postural hypotension, L-dopa can also enhance the effect of co-administered antihypertensive drugs, and blood pressure should be carefully monitored in treated hypertensive patients. Occasionally it may be necessary to advise patients to take antihypertensive medications before bedtime rather than first thing in the morning.

The therapeutic effect of neuroleptic treatment for psychoses may be antagonised by the introduction of L-dopa, and it is advisable that patients requiring neuroleptic medication and therapy for parkinsonian symptoms should be treated with atypical neuroleptics under the guidance of psychiatry and neurology specialist follow-up (*see also Q. 6.13*).

5.22 Is L-dopa safe in pregnancy and breast-feeding?

Probably yes, but there are limited data on this.

Although women of child-bearing age rarely develop parkinsonian syndromes, Parkinson's disease has occurred in women who had not yet completed their families. The limited data available from the literature of seven successful pregnancies while patients were taking Sinemet suggests that this should be the drug of choice in this situation. During the puerperium, treatment with dopamine agonists inhibits prolactin release from the pituitary and therefore decreases milk production in a lactating woman. From the limited information available, this does not seem to occur following L-dopa therapy, and the breast milk produced contains minimal levels of L-dopa. Therefore L-dopa would appear to be a safe drug during breast-feeding. There is little information about the safety of dopamine agonists in pregnancy, and the patient should be counselled regarding benefits of therapy versus possible unknown risks to the fetus.

5.23 Can I combine L-dopa with dopamine agonists?

Yes, and this is often a useful and effective combination.

The majority of patients should nowadays be started on a dopamine agonist, and Sinemet or Madopar should be introduced as an additional agent as soon as the agonist is failing to control the patient's symptoms despite adequate dosage. It is normally recommended that when adding L-dopa, it should be started in a low dose with a simple regime. Both drugs can then be titrated to improve and maximise the patient's response. This practice keeps the dose of L-dopa reasonably low and thus minimises the risk of dyskinesias. It is common practice to use both L-dopa and dopamine agonists at the same time in patients who are not receiving good levels of control despite adequate drug dosing, irrespective of which agent they were first started on.

5.24   What are the monoamine oxidase inhibitors and how do they work?

Drugs such as selegiline that reduce the breakdown of dopamine that is produced either endogenously or after conversion from L-dopa tablets. Monoamine oxidase (MAO) is an enzyme that breaks down dopamine along with other neurotransmitters in the brain. Therefore inhibition of this enzyme will increase the availability of dopamine within the brain, either that which is produced normally or that which is produced by conversion from orally administered L-dopa. The drug which is currently marketed as this is selegiline (an MAO-B inhibitor). Thus this drug is effective in decreasing the metabolism of dopamine and thereby improving its efficacy. It can therefore be useful in the treatment of 'on/off' phenomena by prolonging the effect of L-dopa (*see Ch. 7*).

5.25   Is selegiline protective against the progression of Parkinson's disease?

No.

In the 1980s, a group of drug addicts developed parkinsonism as a result of a toxin accidentally contaminating their heroin. This toxin was identified as MPTP which is toxic to dopamine cells through its conversion to a substance called MPP^+, a conversion that is catalysed by the enzyme monoamine oxidase. It was therefore hypothesised that if Parkinson's disease were due to a similar environmental toxin, which was metabolised by the same enzyme, then inhibiting the enzyme should delay the production of this toxin and thus the development of the disease. A large study was therefore undertaken in the United States, called the DATATOP study in which newly diagnosed patients with Parkinson's disease were randomised to receive a placebo, vitamin E or selegiline. The end point of this trial was the length of time it took until a patient required L-dopa therapy, and it was found that patients put onto selegiline went longer before requiring L-dopa than those on other treatments. Further follow-up and analysis, however, have shown that patients receiving selegiline were receiving symptomatic benefit from the drug rather than being protected against the progression of the disease.

5.26   Was there not a UK trial that showed that selegiline was dangerous to use in Parkinson's disease?

Yes, but re-analysis of the data suggests that the effect was a statistical quirk, and not a real danger.

In 1995, the results of a randomised controlled trial (PDRG-UK) comparing L-dopa treatment with L-dopa/selegiline combination treatment suggested that overall mortality was higher in patients treated with the combination, which led to the drug being discontinued in thousands of patients. Subsequent studies and meta-analyses have not confirmed higher mortality rates in patients taking selegiline, but do not suggest any long-term benefit from early treatment with the drug. Other MAO-B inhibitors have been developed and are being evaluated.

5.27 When should selegiline be used?

Probably when L-dopa fails to produce continuous benefit until the next tablet is due.

There is no evidence that early treatment with selegiline offers long-term benefit; therefore newly diagnosed patients should not necessarily be started on this drug. Selegiline may, however, have a role in the treatment of patients with more advanced disease (*see Q. 7.8*), and there is not sufficient evidence to suggest that stopping the drug in patients that have had long-term good control of symptoms is of benefit. Furthermore, patients who experience a loss of function following withdrawal of selegiline should have the drug re-instituted.

5.28 Are anticholinergic drugs useful as initial treatment?

In some occasional cases, typically in younger patients with tremor-dominant disease.

Initial single therapy with an anticholinergic drug is still very popular with many Parkinson's disease specialists. Anecdotal reports suggest that young patients with hemi-parkinsonism and either tremor or rigidity as the main motor symptom gain the most benefit. The main limitations of these drugs are memory impairment and confusion, particularly in older patients and in those with pre-existing intellectual impairment, in whom these drugs should be avoided. Combination therapy with L-dopa preparations is not advised since this may worsen their psychiatric side-effects, and so in patients needing L-dopa, anticholinergics should be withdrawn gradually after a patient's L-dopa dose has been stabilised. The most commonly used anticholinergic drugs are benzhexol, orphenadrine, benzatropine and biperiden.

5.29 Are β-blockers useful in Parkinson's disease?

Rarely, but they can be of use in patients with bad tremor and profuse sweating.

Propranolol has been used with good effect to ameliorate tremor in patients with anxiety or benign essential tremor. Many Parkinson's disease patients find that their tremor is worsened in public places or during times of anxiety, and in this group of patients propranolol can be useful, either alone or combined with other anti-parkinsonian drugs. Furthermore, propranolol has also been found to help PD patients with episodes of excessive sweating, presumably because of autonomic involvement in the disease process. The more cardioselective β-blockers such as atenolol do not have a beneficial effect on tremor. β-blockers should of course be avoided or used with caution in patients with asthma, cardiac impairment, or peripheral vascular disease.

5.30   What are COMT inhibitors and when should they be used?

Inhibitors of the enzyme that breaks down dopamine.

Catechol-O-methyl transferase (COMT) is an enzyme that metabolises dopamine in the periphery. In the early stages of PD treatment, regular doses of L-dopa produce a sustained benefit in symptoms, whereas in the later stages of disease, a patient's symptoms may fluctuate relative to the timing of L-dopa treatment. COMT inhibitors can be useful in helping the fluctuating symptoms that can be seen in advanced Parkinson's disease (*see* Q. 7.9).

Will I need to take tablets for the rest of my life?

Unfortunately, there are no treatments that can cure or prevent PD. All currently available treatments simply act to alleviate the symptoms of the disease. Since PD is a progressive disease, it is likely that you will need gradually increasing doses of drugs (possibly in combination) from one year to the next. Some patients with advanced disease may be suitable for surgical procedures (*see Ch. 8*), following which drug therapy may be partially, but rarely completely reduced, but your symptoms are certainly not severe enough to warrant a surgical procedure at the moment.

Are you not going to give me a prescription now?

The finding that your symptoms are being caused by Parkinson's disease does not mean that treatment for it has to be started straight away. The first step is to discuss the extent to which your symptoms are interfering with your lifestyle. You will certainly need to start treatment at some point, and you will probably need to have increases in your medication from time to time to keep your symptoms under control. Unfortunately, prolonged treatment with anti-Parkinson drugs tends to lead to side-effects after a number of years, and for this reason it is not advisable to start taking tablets until your symptoms are either causing you inconvenience or affecting your lifestyle.

How soon will I notice a benefit from taking tablets?

The length of time before you notice any improvement varies from patient to patient but the majority of people who benefit from anti-Parkinson's tablets will notice some improvement in their symptoms within the first month. For some people, the improvements that they notice are quite small while they are taking low doses of tablets, and the dose may need to be increased several times before you get the maximum benefit. In addition, some people do not 'get on' with the first drug that is tried, and it may be necessary to try several drugs before finding the combination to best suit you.

Do these tablets have any side-effects?

Unfortunately, all tablets have side-effects, but most of these are either mild or affect only a minority of people. The main side-effects that occur with the anti-Parkinson's medications are a feeling of *nausea* (which can be minimised by taking your tablets with food) or *dizziness* due to the blood pressure falling when you stand up quickly. Your blood pressure will be monitored at each visit to the surgery/clinic.

Taking L-dopa tablets for many years can cause some people to have abnormal additional movements which we call *dyskinesias*. These movements do eventually occur in all people and can be controlled initially by slight changes in dosage. The newer tablets for Parkinson's disease cause these movements much less frequently and so we tend to use these first of all. There is also a long list of possible side-effects on the information sheet that comes with the tablets; however, most of these are very rare indeed, and should not deter you from taking the tablets. (*See also Qs 5.9 and 5.19.*)

My friend has Parkinson's disease and her tablets are different from mine. Why?

There are now a large variety of tablets that are used to treat Parkinson's disease. Some of these tablets work in similar ways to each other but they are manufactured by different drug companies and are therefore called different names. From the research trials that have been done, it has been shown that many of these tablets are just as good as each other; therefore if your symptoms are well controlled on one, you should stay on it. If your symptoms are not so well controlled, then either the dose should be increased or a different tablet should be tried. Also, some patients feel better on one tablet compared to others, and that may be why your friend is on different medication.

What is the difference between Sinemet and Madopar?

Sinemet and Madopar contain exactly the same active drug to help the symptoms of Parkinson's disease. This drug is called L-dopa. Both types of tablet also contain a second chemical which helps minimise the side-effects such as sickness that can occur with L-dopa. The second chemicals are slightly different in Sinemet and Madopar, which is the only difference between them. If you find one of these tablets unpleasant, you may find that the other one suits you better.

What is a dopamine agonist?

Dopamine agonists are types of drugs that are able to mimic the effects of dopamine by stimulating the same parts of the brain. They can relieve your symptoms of Parkinson's disease almost as well as L-dopa, and while they still have some short-term side-effects, the long-term side-effects occur less often than with L-dopa.

What is the best treatment for Parkinson's disease?

The best treatment for Parkinson's disease varies from one individual to the next. There are several different types of tablet that may all have some effect in relieving your symptoms. Unfortunately, all tablets have some side-effects, and it is necessary to decide which tablet will have the most benefit for your specific symptoms while not causing these unpleasant side-effects. In addition, it is necessary to think about the future, and make sure that your treatment is sufficient to keep your quality of life good now, but not so much that it causes you to have long-term side-effects.

Drug treatment of Parkinson's disease (non-motor symptoms)

6

6.1 What are the non-motor symptoms of Parkinson's disease?

See Box 6.1.

BOX 6.1 Non-motor symptoms seen in some patients with PD

- Salivary drooling
- Sweating and seborrhoea
- Constipation
- Bladder instability
- Postural hypotension
- Sleep disturbance
- Cognitive impairment
- Depression

6.2 Are there drugs which help with salivary drooling?

 Yes, but side-effects may occur.

 Many patients with Parkinson's disease have abnormalities of saliva production and swallowing. For patients with salivary drooling (*sialorrhoea*), a useful side-effect of the anticholinergic drugs is a reduction in saliva production. Many patients and especially the elderly are, however, intolerant of centrally acting anticholinergic agents because of memory impairment, confusion or hallucinations. For these patients, peripherally acting anticholinergics such as propantheline are the preferred treatments in reducing salivary drooling. Other treatments that may be used are hyoscine patches or botulinus toxin injections. In extreme cases, where these simple measures fail, patients may benefit from parotid irradiation to block saliva production, although this should be viewed as a last desperate resort.

Occasionally patients complain of reduced saliva production. In these cases it is important to exclude drugs as a cause of this, and ensure that the patient does not have any other explanation for a dry mouth, such as Sjögren's syndrome. Unfortunately, if no cause can be found, the only advice that can be given is to eat with plenty of fluids and to encourage salivary production with the sucking of sweets.

6.3 Do any drugs help with sweating or seborrhoea?

Yes, β-blockers or modifying L-dopa regimes may help.

Severe sweats can occur as a dose of L-dopa wears off, and increasing the frequency of L-dopa dosing or controlled-release agents may be of benefit to such patients. Some patients, however, experience sweating in response to a dose of L-dopa and may require a reduction in dosing, titrated in accordance with their motor symptoms. These patients are also more likely to benefit from β-blockers such as propranolol than are patients with 'off'-period sweating.

Daily application of topical hydrocortisone may be effective for excessive seborrhoea occurring on the face, and if this is not effective topical ketoconazole is an alternative. Coal tar shampoos can be used for seborrhoea developing over the eyebrows and forehead.

6.4 What is the treatment for constipation in Parkinson's disease?

The usual therapies.

Constipation is a very common symptom among Parkinson's disease patients and is often overlooked. In the first instance, patients with mild constipation should be advised to increase their intake of fibre and attempt to increase exercise levels (*see also Ch. 9*). Anticholinergic therapies can also contribute to slowed bowel transit, and dose reduction or cessation of these may increase bowel motility. Patients with more severe constipation should be treated judiciously with stool softeners, laxatives or enemas prior to the use of gut stimulants. Apomorphine can also be used as a rescue for severe constipation during 'off' periods (*see Q. 7.17*). Whilst constipation is common in PD, it is obviously important to ensure that the constipation is due to PD and that other causes have not been overlooked.

6.5 What is the best treatment for bladder instability in Parkinson's disease?

Exclude other causes, and then consider oxybutynin.

A change in the voiding pattern of a Parkinson's disease patient should always prompt a search for a possible urinary tract infection, and in male patients it is always important to remember prostatism as a cause for bladder symptoms. If symptoms of frequency or urgency persist in the absence of infection or prostatism, urological investigation can distinguish between detrusor hyperactivity and hypoactivity. It is important to make sure, of course, that the symptoms do not relate to drugs that the patient may be taking, e.g. anticholinergics.

Detrusor hyperactivity should be treated with peripherally acting anticholinergics such as oxybutynin or propantheline. PD patients with hypoactive detrusor muscles should not be given α-blocking agents such as prazosin since they can induce severe orthostatic hypotension. Intermittent catheterisation may be the best treatment for patients with overdistended hypoactive bladders.

Bladder symptoms may also occur as a symptom of multiple system atrophy, one of the Parkinson-plus disorders (*see Ch. 10*). If patients have prominent bladder symptoms early on in the course of their parkinsonian illness, then this should alert the clinician to the possibility that the patient is developing MSA. In such cases, a search for other signs of autonomic failure such as marked postural hypotension or erectile dysfunction should be made (*Box 6.2*).

BOX 6.2 Features of autonomic failure

■ Postural hypotension
■ Impotence
■ Urinary incontinence or retention
■ Loss of sweating

6.6 What is the best treatment for postural hypotension in Parkinson's disease?

Simple measures, e.g. head-up bed tilt, or fludrocortisone.

Postural hypotension can usually be diagnosed on the basis of a clear history of dizziness on standing; however, it may take several minutes of standing for blood pressure to fall. This should be remembered when postural blood pressure measurements are being made. Parkinson's disease patients with autonomic involvement causing postural hypotension are not uncommon, and these patients should avoid antihypertensive medications. Drugs such as the dopamine agonists and L-dopa should be introduced gradually to minimise their hypotensive side-effects. If such symptoms occur early in the course of the illness and are marked, then it is possible that the patient is developing MSA rather than having PD.

In the first instance, management involves simple advice. The patient should be told to stand up slowly to minimise the risk of falling and patients and their families should be educated about the hypotensive effects of food, hot weather, and physical exertion. PD patients with autonomic failure should eat frequent small meals with low carbohydrate content and avoid alcoholic beverages. Hot baths also can induce hypotension and should be avoided.

Other simple measures such as elevating the head of the bed and using full-length compression stockings may also be helpful if tolerated. If necessary, fludrocortisone 0.1–0.5 mg/day, or intranasal DDAVP 5–40 μg may improve symptoms by increasing intravascular circulating blood volume. In practice, the best management involves a combination of education, head-up (*not* feet-up) bed tilt, and a low dose of fludrocortisone. More aggressive treatment requires specialist input and involves using sympathomimetic agents, e.g. midodrine, to increase peripheral vascular resistance. The blood pressure response to midodrine occurs within hours of an oral dose, and therapy is usually started at a dose of 2.5 mg and is increased to no more than 10 mg t.d.s.

6.7 Are there any treatments for sleep disturbance in Parkinson's disease?

Yes, but it depends on the underlying cause.

The major causes of sleep disturbances in Parkinson's disease patients are insomnia, nightmares or restless legs, and may relate to drug therapy, PD or the development of a dementia (*Table 6.1*).

Poorly controlled parkinsonian features such as tremor, or inability to turn over in bed also cause insomnia and can be alleviated with long-acting dopaminergic preparations, dopamine agonists taken last thing at night or COMT inhibitors (*see Q. 7.9*). Insomnia also commonly occurs following the introduction of dopaminergic medication, but this is usually a transient phenomenon and sedative medications are usually not required. Short-acting sedatives can be useful for insomnia that persists independently of changes in anti-PD medication, but physical dependence or cognitive impairment may occur. In cases in which benzodiazepines are not effective, tricyclic antidepressants may be used cautiously but have the risk of precipitating confusion or hallucinations.

L-dopa-induced dyskinesias preventing sleep require a reduction in night-time L-dopa or dopamine agonist dose. Depression or anxiety should always be considered in patients with PD as a cause for their insomnia.

Nightmares may also occur secondary to dopaminergic medication and may herald the onset of a dopaminergic psychosis or signify a developing dementia. Reduction of night-time L-dopa, or the introduction of an atypical neuroleptic (*see Q. 6.13*) may be necessary.

Restless legs may be idiopathic in origin or may be a symptom of PD (*see Q. 2.17*). In either case, symptoms are relieved by dopaminergic medication. In patients resistant to such treatment, clonazepam, gabapentin or clonidine may be useful, and consideration should be given to the possibility that their RLS may be due to some other cause. Tricyclic antidepressants should be avoided as these may worsen the condition.

It is clearly also important to give consideration to the possibility that other primary sleep disturbances can occur in PD and include REM sleep behaviour disorder (RSBD) or obstructive sleep apnoea. Where there is confusion regarding the cause of sleep disturbance, sleep tests (polysomnography) should be performed at specialist centres.

Daytime drowsiness has rarely been described following each dose of L-dopa and more recently has been linked to certain dopamine agonists (*see Q. 5.10*). Such symptoms and problems can usually be resolved by adjustment of the amount and timing of each dose. Stimulatory drugs to relieve daytime drowsiness are generally not necessary, but caffeine or even amfetamine preparations have been required, although they are not recommended without advice from specialist clinics. Patients with daytime drowsiness should be questioned about sleep attacks and advised not to drive.

TABLE 6.1 Diagnosis and treatment of sleep disturbance in PD

Sleep disturbance	Cause	Treatment
Insomnia	1. Uncontrolled symptoms of PD as evidenced by inability to turn over or get out of bed	Increase PD medication – slow-release L-dopa medication or dopamine agonist last thing at night
	2. Introduction of new dopamine agonist	Encourage persistence with medication
	3. Uncontrolled dyskinesias	Reduce night-time dopamine medication
	4. Depression/anxiety	Treat depression or anxiety
Nightmares	1. Excess dopaminergic medication	Reduce dopaminergic medication
	2. Underlying cortical involvement in disease process	Treat as in Figure 6.1
Restless legs	Undertreated PD	Increase dopaminergic medication
	RLS is not uncommonly seen in PD, although it is also seen in a range of other conditions such as anaemia and renal failure (*see Q. 2.17*)	Consider trials of benzodiazepines, opioids, clonazepam, gabapentin or clonidine, all of which have been described to help this condition
Other sleep disturbances*	1. REM sleep behaviour disorder	Clonazepam
	2. Obstructive sleep apnoea	Weight loss, assisted ventilation
	3. Nocturia	Investigation and treatment as in Question 6.5

* These other sleep disorders can normally only be diagnosed in specialist sleep clinics, and referral is advised if there is doubt regarding the nature of the sleep disturbance.

6.8 Can cognitive impairment in Parkinson's disease be treated?

Yes, by minimising causative factors and using atypical neuroleptics or cholinesterase inhibitors (*Fig. 6.1*).

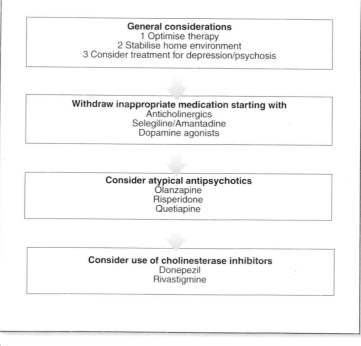

Fig. 6.1 Approach to the management of cognitive impairment in PD.

Most medical therapies in Parkinson's disease aim to improve the motor symptoms of the disease. However, it is clear that treatment to optimise motor symptoms can also improve cognitive impairment. It is also clear that these medications can make things worse from a cognitive perspective and that some drugs are especially prone to causing these problems. Therefore one way of improving a patient's cognitive state is by re-evaluating and modifying the patient's drug therapy for PD. Certain medications should be avoided in susceptible patients (e.g. anticholinergics in the elderly). Further improvement of cognitive function may also result from addressing other contributing factors such as depression, and the maintenance of a stable home environment.

In addition, some results have shown that atypical neuroleptics such as quetiapine and clozapine may indeed improve cognitive performance in PD patients, without worsening their PD. However, these drugs should only (and in the case of clozapine, *can* only) be prescribed by specialist clinics. Finally, there are ongoing trials investigating the potential use of cholinesterase inhibitors such as donepezil and rivastigmine. These are licensed in Alzheimer's dementia and have been shown to be beneficial in dementia with Lewy bodies, and so may become more widely used in patients with cognitive impairment in PD.

6.9 How do I treat Parkinson's disease patients with acute confusion?

By looking for an underlying cause as for any confused patient.

Table 6.2 outlines a general approach to treating confusion, with specific reference to Parkinson's disease patients. In essence, a cause should be sought and treated. However, even when aetiological agents (e.g. UTIs) have been identified and treated, the patient may still remain confused. In these circumstances, the gradual cessation of adjunctive treatments

TABLE 6.2 Approach to the management of acute confusional states in PD patients

Has there been a change in the patient's environment?	Attempt to stabilise the patient's environment. Avoid unfamiliar settings and ensure good lighting
Is there an underlying, treatable medical cause?	Exclude infection in chest, urine or skin sites. Perform blood tests to assess metabolic derangement. If fluctuating consciousness or head injury – consider subdural haemorrhage, meningitis or encephalitis
Has there been a recent alteration in medication?	Withdraw any new anti-parkinsonian medications, or tricyclic antidepressants
Is the patient excessively agitated?	Consider use of sedative short term
Is confusion becoming prolonged?	Reduce adjunctive anti-parkinsonian medications (anticholinergics, amantadine, COMT inhibitors, dopamine agonists)
Situation not improving despite above measures?	Consider atypical neuroleptic

(e.g. anticholinergics then dopaminergic agonists) over a couple of weeks followed by reduction of L-dopa dose should be attempted prior to commencing an atypical neuroleptic. Agents such as olanzapine, risperidone, and quetiapine have been shown to be helpful and benzodiazepine sedatives such as lorazepam may be required in the short term if there is distressing agitation.

6.10 What treatments are available for depression in Parkinson's disease?

 The same as for any other depressed patients (*Table 6.3*).

 Symptoms of parkinsonism may be accompanied by a reactive depressive state that may be lifted following treatment of the disease. In addition, therapy may lead to an improvement of facial masking (hypomimia), thus making a patient appear to be more cheerful.

True depression associated with Parkinson's disease often responds to tricyclic antidepressants, which can also help patients with difficulty sleeping, owing to their soporific effects. The anticholinergic side-effects of tricyclics may also provide some benefit to their parkinsonian symptoms, although they may lead to worsening of confusion, especially in the elderly, as well as dry mouth and urinary symptoms.

Selective serotonin reuptake inhibitors (SSRIs) are also effective agents but may aggravate parkinsonian motor symptoms if anti-Parkinson drugs are not being used simultaneously. SSRIs may also interact with certain drugs, e.g. selegiline, which precludes their use. Some newer antidepressants have combined selective serotonin reuptake inhibitory activity with either noradrenaline (norepinephrine) reuptake inhibition (venlafaxine) or serotonergic antagonism (nefazodone). These agents have shown promising results in the treatment of depression in the general population but have not undergone any formal trials in PD. Electroconvulsive therapy (ECT) can help patients with intractable depression, and can also transiently improve the motor symptoms of the disease. However, decisions regarding such treatments require the involvement of experienced psychiatrists.

6.11 Are there any problems in commencing an antidepressant in Parkinson's disease?

 Usually not, if side-effect profiles are taken into account.

Very few well-constructed trials investigating the individual effects of antidepressants in Parkinson's disease have been conducted, and for this

TABLE 6.3 Common antidepressant medications used in PD

	Tricyclic antidepressants (TCAs) and related treatments	Selective serotonin reuptake inhibitors (SSRIs)	Monoamine oxidase inhibitors (MAOI-As)
Preparations	Amitriptyline Imipramine Trazodone	Fluoxetine Sertraline Paroxetine	Phenelzine Moclobemide
Effectiveness	A lot of experience with their use, and a small number of controlled trials showing benefit in PD whilst not exacerbating motor symptoms	Open label studies showed good effectiveness but a low risk of exacerbating motor symptoms	Not usually first line but have been shown to be beneficial. Occasional benefit for motor symptoms
Side-effects	Anticholinergic Confusion (should be avoided in those patients on trihexyphenidyl (benzhexol), procyclidine) Drowsiness Dry mouth Blurred vision Constipation Urinary retention Cardiovascular – Arrhythmias – Heart block	Less sedating and cardiotoxic than TCAs Minor disturbances (e.g. nausea, diarrhoea, rash, headache) Low risk of exacerbating extrapyramidal motor features and dyskinesias Exceedingly rare 'serotonin syndrome' hypersensitivity type reaction*	Through their action, MAOIs cause build-up of amine neurotransmitters, which may precipitate dangerous hypertension Need to avoid tyramine-rich foods (e.g. cheese, Bovril, Marmite) and cough/decongestant preparations

*The serotonin syndrome is a potentially serious drug-related condition characterised by confusion, agitation, tachycardia, sweating and hyperpyrexia. Some patients may require admission to ITU.

reason most common practice is based on personal experiences. Decisions on the appropriate timing and choice of an antidepressant must always be taken based on the individual case. The main limitation of any of the antidepressants is the side-effect profile associated with the drug. Deterioration in PD symptoms following the introduction of an SSRI tends to improve after withdrawal of the drug, and many PD specialists now use these drugs as their first choice for the treatment of depression in PD.

6.12   What is the best treatment for anxiety in Parkinson's disease?

Benzodiazepines, but anxiety may relate to the control of PD symptoms.

Benzodiazepines are the most commonly used drugs to improve anxiety symptoms, of which lorazepam is usually well tolerated in older patients, whereas diazepam and chlordiazepoxide are usually less well tolerated. β-blockers may be useful for anxiety-related tachycardia. Barbiturates should be avoided. In some cases, the anxiety is related to the disease and its control. Education and support can help, and in those patients who have anxious 'off' periods, attention should be paid to improving their motor control with standard anti-PD drugs.

6.13   What is the treatment for hallucinations and psychosis in Parkinson's disease?

Modifying the anti-PD drug regime and using atypical antipsychotics.

If hallucinations are a prominent symptom in the early stages of a parkinsonian syndrome, the diagnosis of dementia with Lewy bodies (DLB) should be considered (*see Q. 3.3*). It is possible that the introduction of an acetylcholinesterase inhibitor such as donepezil or rivastigmine may be useful for patients with DLB in the future.

Patients with established, typical Parkinson's disease who develop hallucinations or psychosis should be assessed in a logical manner. Triggering factors such as infections, metabolic disorders and other hallucinogenic drugs should be excluded in the same way as for acutely confused patients. The second step is to eliminate anti-parkinsonian drugs in the following order: anticholinergics, selegiline, amantadine, dopamine agonists and then L-dopa itself. While reducing the dosage of such medications may benefit behavioural symptoms, this is usually accompanied by deterioration in physical function. As such, a balance may be needed, taking into account the level of mobility desired by the patient and the hazards of psychosis for both patient and carers. Temporary admission to hospital may be necessary in this situation, although it can worsen the situation as a result of changing environments.

If psychotic episodes persist despite minimising anti-PD treatments, or unacceptable levels of disability from the PD occur, antipsychotic drugs should be considered. The classical neuroleptic medications are to be avoided in patients suffering with PD, as owing to their dopamine antagonist actions, they will worsen PD symptoms. Newer, atypical neuroleptic medications (e.g. clozapine, olanzapine, risperidone, quetiapine) have been developed, which have less of these problematic physical side-effects, although are not without side-effects themselves (*see Table 6.4*). These drugs act less as dopamine D_2-receptor antagonists and more by serotonin $5\text{-}HT_2$-receptor antagonism. This therapeutic approach has led to some very successful results with improvement in patient symptoms without deterioration in physical function and makes these agents the popular choice in the management of PD patients.

This new generation of antipsychotic medication are, however, generally quite expensive treatments and require close patient observation. Most of these agents are sedating, which is undesirable, and clozapine has been found to cause agranulocytosis in about 1% of cases. This has led to its prescription only by authorised centres and demands stringent patient monitoring with blood tests.

TABLE 6.4 The atypical neuroleptic drugs

Drug	Indication	Mechanism of action	Side-effects
Clozapine	Anxiety Depression Hypersexuality Sleep disturbance Akathisia	D_1, D_3 and D_4 antagonist	Sedation Granulocytopenia Agranulocytosis
Risperidone	L-dopa-induced hallucinations	$5\text{-}HT_2$ antagonist D_2 antagonist	Deterioration in PD symptoms
Olanzapine	Psychotic symptoms in PD	$5\text{-}HT_{2A/2C}$ antagonist D_1, D_2, D_4 antagonist	Sedation Dry mouth Weight gain Deranged liver function tests Deterioration in PD symptoms
Quetiapine	Psychotic symptoms in PD	$5\text{-}HT_2$ antagonist D_2 antagonist	Little information to date

PQ PATIENT QUESTIONS

Could those tablets you gave me have made me start seeing things?

Occasionally people do suffer from confusion or even hallucinations with medications used for Parkinson's disease. If this occurs, you should stop taking the prescribed tablets. There are other similar preparations that can be tried instead, and you will be given a very low dose to start with. If you do have problems again, stop the tablets immediately and see your doctor.

My Parkinson's disease is much better but can you give me something to help me sleep?

It is not unusual for people to have trouble sleeping as the dose of their tablets is increased. This usually passes within a week or two of reaching a stable dose. It is therefore preferable not to prescribe a course of sleeping tablets at a time when your natural sleep pattern should be returning, and sleeping tablets might prolong the problem if you start to rely on them. However, if sleep continues to be a problem, it may be necessary to reconsider this.

He gets so confused on these tablets, is there anything that can be done to help?

In the first instance, it will be necessary to do a few medical tests to make sure that there are no other problems causing his confusion. If the confusion is definitely due to the tablets, then the dose should be reduced. If there is no improvement after this, the tablets should be stopped completely. If the symptoms of Parkinson's disease become uncontrolled on a lower dose, then alternative tablets should be considered. At the same time, it is important to ensure that he has a familiar routine and environment at home.

I seem to be drooling the whole time, it's so embarrassing – is there anything that helps?

It can be hard to stop the increased saliva production that is caused by Parkinson's disease. The first treatment to try is a tablet called propantheline, which should reduce the amount of saliva that you produce. If this does not work, there are other things that can be tried, such as patches, or you may be suitable for injections into the salivary glands themselves.

Complications of Parkinson's disease and treatment of advanced disease

7

7.1 What is advanced Parkinson's disease?

It signifies patients with variable responses to treatment or complications from their treatments, usually after many years of the condition.

'Advanced Parkinson's disease' refers to patients who have entered the complex treatment phase of the disease (*see Q. 1.26*). Patients describe variation in their symptoms during the course of the day, and suffer from complications related to the treatments they are receiving. Patients with advanced PD require adjustments of the dose and timing of their tablets to minimise these complications.

7.2 What complications occur in patients with advanced Parkinson's disease?

 Dyskinesias, unpredictable responses to drugs, confusion, hallucinations and falls.

 Prolonged treatment with L-dopa almost inevitably leads to side-effects such as dyskinesias, dystonia or hallucinations (*Table 7.1*). In addition, patients may have a decline in the benefit they receive from L-dopa, leading to motor or cognitive fluctuations. It is still controversial whether these adverse outcomes are due to worsening of the underlying disease or due to the sustained use of L-dopa, but on average 10% of patients per year of treatment develop complications.

TABLE 7.1 Complications seen in advanced PD

Complication	Subtypes
Fluctuations	'Wearing off' 'On-off' phenomenon Delayed 'on' or no 'on' Freezing episodes
Dyskinesias	Peak dose End of dose Biphasic

7.3 What are 'on/off' fluctuations?

Motor responses to treatment in Parkinson's disease, with 'on' being free of parkinsonian symptoms and 'off' being the state where parkinsonian symptoms have re-emerged.

Motor 'on/off' fluctuations refer to the variation in the severity of symptoms (*Table 7.2 and Fig. 7.1*) and are most frequent in patients treated with L-dopa. Fluctuations usually begin as mild '*wearing off*' episodes in which a patient feels that the improvement gained from a dose of medication gradually diminishes and does not last until the time that the next dose is due. Subsequently, fluctuations then progress to 'on' periods of good symptom control following a dose of L-dopa, followed by 'off' periods as the parkinsonian symptoms re-emerge, either partially or completely. These 'off' periods can become quite unpredictable. 'On' periods can also be characterised by the development of additional involuntary movements termed dyskinesias (*see Q. 7.11*). Fluctuations in motor symptoms are the most common, but mood and autonomic functions may also fluctuate in parallel with these motor symptoms. 'Non-motor off periods' are usually milder than 'motor off periods' but can lead to unnecessary tests or prescriptions if not recognised. Fluctuations may rarely occur in a patient naive to dopaminergic drugs. The mechanism underlying this is not clear.

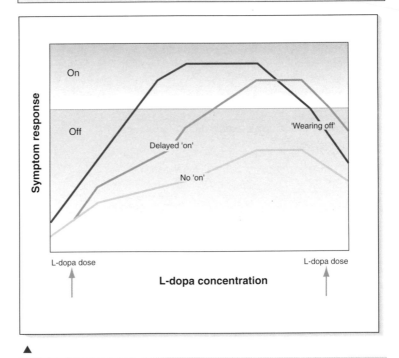

Fig. 7.1 Graphical representation of motor fluctuations seen in PD.

TABLE 7.2 Motor fluctuations seen in advanced PD

Fluctuation	Timing
'Wearing off'	End of dose return of PD symptoms
'On/off' phenomenon	Unpredictable return of symptoms during response to drug dose
Delayed 'on' or no 'on'	Dose fails to relieve symptoms at all or only after delay
Freezing episodes	Unpredictable

7.4 What causes 'on/off' fluctuations?

Not known, but probably relates to erratic uptake of L-dopa in gut and brain.

It is still unresolved as to what causes fluctuations in a patient's response to L-dopa. It is known that as the disease progresses the number of nerve terminals remaining in the nigrostriatal tract becomes smaller, and the uptake of L-dopa becomes more critical in governing the response. The uptake of L-dopa across the gut and brain, and ultimately into the nerve terminals, is somewhat erratic and there are many other compounds or proteins which compete for uptake into these sites. It is therefore thought that in the early stages of the disease, there are enough nerve terminals present to ensure that there is a buffering of this erratic uptake to produce a relatively smooth motor response. However, as the disease progresses and the number of terminals declines, the erratic response becomes more manifest with either no L-dopa being taken up, which produces the 'off' state, or excessive amounts taken up and released as dopamine, causing dyskinetic movements (see Q. 7.11). However, having said this, it is highly probable that the reality is even more complex and subtle than this and that there are also changes within the striatum itself with alterations in receptor properties and effects.

7.5 What is freezing?

Sudden 'off' periods causing patients to stick to the spot.

Freezing usually describes a sudden 'off period'. This is most often seen during walking as 'start hesitation', 'turning hesitation' or 'sudden freezing' as if the feet are glued to the floor. Often the latter occurs when patients are confronted by narrow spaces, e.g. doorways.

7.6 What causes freezing?

Not known.

Freezing is a type of motor fluctuation but the underlying cause of this phenomenon is not known. 'Off' freezing can be thought of as a feature of

Parkinson's disease and is best treated by keeping the patient switched 'on'. Freezing can, however, also occur during 'on' periods, which is more difficult both to explain and to treat, since increasing the dosage of L-dopa tends to aggravate the problem. Patients can, however, use various physical tricks to overcome this type of freezing and these are described in Chapter 9 (*see* Q. 9.7).

7.7 Can patient diaries be helpful?

Yes, provided the patient does not become too introspective.

Difficulty interpreting a patient's pattern of symptoms can be more facilitated in a short consultation if patients keep a diary to record times of day that they have good symptom control, times that they become more parkinsonian and times that they experience dyskinesias.

Diaries can, however, occasionally lead to severe introspection of patients considering their symptoms. This can be counterproductive and may lead to patients changing their treatment on a daily basis, which makes it impossible to advise on treatment.

7.8 How can I treat motor fluctuations?

Establish an accurate description of fluctuations and modify the drug regime to reduce 'off' periods and increase 'on' time.

At first 'on/off' fluctuations are predictable and can usually be improved by taking more frequent, smaller doses of L-dopa. Some patients, however, progress to a situation where fluctuations are unpredictable and can occur quite suddenly. In this situation the patient may prefer to return to less-frequent, higher doses of L-dopa, resulting in longer 'off' periods but enabling the 'on' periods to be more reliably symptom free. Patients with unpredictable 'offs' may also benefit from a redistribution or lowering of protein in their diet (*see* Q. 9.11).

Treatment of 'on/off' fluctuations becomes more complicated if the 'on' periods are accompanied by the development of dyskinetic movements. Patients may, however, prefer to tolerate dyskinetic movements during 'on' periods rather than have excessive 'off' time. Alternative strategies to treat fluctuations are the use of entacapone (*see* Q. 7.9) or selegiline (*see* Q. 5.27).

7.9 What is entacapone?

An inhibitor of the enzyme that breaks down dopamine, so promoting its effectiveness.

In addition to metabolism by amino acid decarboxylase, L-dopa is also metabolised by the catechol-O-methyl transferase (COMT) enzyme. Entacapone (Comtess) inhibits this enzyme, and thus extends the plasma half-life of L-dopa. It appears to be useful for treating fluctuations following prolonged L-dopa therapy and allows the dose of L-dopa to be reduced.

Needless to say, because of the increased availability of L-dopa following initiation of entacapone, nausea, vomiting and increased dyskinesias may be seen, necessitating L-dopa reduction.

Tolcapone (Tasmar) is another inhibitor of the COMT enzyme. This drug has previously been widely used to treat patients with complications of Parkinson's disease. Case reports identified a drug-induced hepatitis that can develop in response to the use of the drug and this has led to the drug being withdrawn in the UK. A very few patients who refused to be taken off the drug, or did not tolerate switching to entacapone, remain on tolcapone within the UK, by getting supplies from sources overseas. Liver function tests should be stringently monitored in these patients, with appropriate support and regular specialist review.

It is also possible that the administration of L-dopa with a COMT inhibitor from the time it is first introduced might reduce the pulsatile nature of dopamine receptor stimulation, and as a result reduce the risk of subsequent motor complications. However, this remains unproven.

7.10 How should entacapone be started?

Slowly, and with L-dopa, following review at specialist clinics.

Entacapone should generally only be started on the basis of specialist advice. The starting dose of entacapone is 200 mg to be taken with each dose of L-dopa, up to a maximum of 8 doses per day. Typically, the L-dopa dose will need to be lowered by about 20% following the introduction of entacapone. Reduction of the L-dopa dose should be done as soon as the new drug is started to prevent the development of side-effects from too much L-dopa, which patients might attribute to the entacapone and subsequently develop a fear of the drug. Patients should be warned that their urine is likely to become discoloured following initiation of treatment with entacapone.

7.11 What are dyskinetic movements?

Abnormal involuntary movements that develop in response to drug treatments in advanced Parkinson's disease.

Dyskinetic movements refer to abnormal movements that are induced by dopaminergic drugs, consisting of dance-like movements involving the arms, legs and trunk. These movements can be so severe that patients begin to wriggle around uncontrollably such that they can even force themselves off chairs, onto the floor, and may risk damage to themselves as their limbs move around abnormally. In some patients, the rapid dance-like movements do not occur, but instead a fixed abnormal posturing of the limbs takes place, so-called dystonia. This later symptom can be difficult to diagnose because it also occurs in the untreated parkinsonian state, and thus its presence may be hard to interpret in terms of whether the patient is under- or overtreated. A careful history regarding the timing of dystonic movements can usually distinguish between 'on dystonia' and 'off dystonia'.

7.12 When do dyskinetic movements occur?

Typically after taking dopaminergic medication, although the timing may vary.

L-dopa-induced dyskinesias very rarely occur early in the course of L-dopa treatment, but are common in patients treated with L-dopa for more than 3–5 years. They most frequently occur at the time of 'peak dose', but are also recognised as an 'end of dose' phenomenon, or occur more rarely as the level of L-dopa is both rising and falling – 'biphasic dyskinesias'.

In patients who are maintained on CR preparations, the dyskinesia may only become apparent towards the end of the day as the dose of L-dopa accumulates.

7.13 What causes dyskinesias?

Abnormal release of dopamine in the brain as a consequence of years of treatment with dopaminergic drugs.

It is now thought that long-term, non-physiological stimulation of striatal dopamine receptors that occurs with *pulsatile* dopaminergic therapy, leads to maladaptive events downstream from the dopamine receptors and it is these that cause these abnormal movements.

As a result, there is increasing interest in drugs to treat this problem that do not work on the dopaminergic system (e.g. the glutamate, adenosine, cannabinoid and opiate systems). However, these still remain at an experimental stage of development. Whatever the explanation, it is probable that there are several abnormalities of basal ganglia function that underlie the generation of different dyskinesias.

7.14 How can I treat dyskinesias?

Treatment is complicated and requires help from specialist clinics.

In the first instance, the early use of dopamine agonists slows the development of dyskinetic movements, in comparison to the frequency with which they are seen with L-dopa therapy. Almost all patients, however, eventually require additional L-dopa therapy and risk the development of dyskinesias. Once dyskinesias have become established, modification of the drug treatment can still help.

PEAK DOSE DYSKINESIAS

If the dyskinetic movements occur at peak dose, i.e. at the midpoint between two doses of Sinemet or Madopar, then it is advised to reduce the dose of medication in 25-mg increments, and perhaps give it more frequently. It is also usually easier to control dyskinesia by switching from the controlled-release to the regular formulation of L-dopa to prevent L-dopa accumulating throughout the day.

One can also try to smooth out the motor response and achieve continuous dopamine receptor stimulation by the use of dopamine agonists, which may also allow a reduction in the L-dopa dose.

Alternatively, the use of potentiators of dopamine, namely the monoamine oxidase inhibitors (*see Q. 5.24*) and the COMT inhibitors (*see Q. 7.9*), may also be helpful in smoothing out responses and reducing dyskinesias. However, it is important to remember that the introduction of a COMT inhibitor to a patient with dyskinesias will cause a worsening of these, unless the L-dopa dose is concomitantly reduced. It has been demonstrated in both animals and humans that attempts to produce continuous stimulation of dopamine receptors with either L-dopa or a dopamine agonist administered subcutaneously can dramatically reduce the frequency and severity of dyskinesias. Antidyskinetic agents (such as amantadine – *see Q. 7.15*) or surgery should be considered in refractory patients.

BIPHASIC DYSKINESIAS

If, on the other hand, the abnormal movements occur just after the treatment is taken and just before it wears off (so-called biphasic dyskinetic movements), then it is advised that the patient takes higher, less-frequent doses of L-dopa in an attempt to provide a more continuous 'on' state and prevent the patient from cycling through the dyskinetic phases. (This pattern of dyskinesia followed by improvement followed by dyskinesia is sometimes referred to as D-I-D dyskinesia.) Addition of a dopamine agonist is usually not helpful for these biphasic dyskinesias, although subcutaneous apomorphine may provide additional 'on' time to sustain the patient until a response is achieved from the next dose of L-dopa.

Addition of amantadine, has also been reported to decrease severity of biphasic dyskinesias without worsening control of parkinsonian symptoms.

7.15 What is amantadine?

An agent that has recently been found to be very useful in treating drug-induced dyskinesias.

Amantadine (Symmetrel) is an anti-influenza drug which has been observed to increase the availability of brain dopamine, and possibly has some anticholinergic and antiglutamatergic actions as well. It is relatively cheap and about two-thirds of Parkinson's disease patients improve on it alone or in combination with L-dopa preparations. It can be useful as initial drug monotherapy (starting at 100 mg daily), although this is now rarely done. However, recently, it has been found to be especially helpful in the management of drug-induced dyskinesias. Typical dose requirements are 200 mg once daily, but the dose may need to be increased to as high as 200 mg twice daily. Amantadine may cause ankle oedema, and hallucinations in patients on higher doses.

7.16 What is the role of dopamine agonists in the later stages of Parkinson's disease?

To improve and smooth out motor symptoms with a reduction in L-dopa requirements.

Dopamine agonists now have an established use in patients with motor fluctuations, dystonia or dyskinesias. They can allow the dose of L-dopa to be lowered, which reduces the dyskinesias, while maintaining patients in an 'on' state. In addition, patients may have a decreasing therapeutic response to L-dopa at advanced stages of disease owing to failure of metabolism of the drug to dopamine by dwindling numbers of presynaptic dopaminergic neurons. Dopamine agonists do not need metabolism and therefore can be effective at the intact postsynaptic dopamine receptors, and can thus help restore control of parkinsonian symptoms. As with early Parkinson's disease, they can be especially helpful in controlling nocturnal symptoms.

7.17 What is apomorphine?

 A non-selective dopamine agonist that can only be given subcutaneously and in combination with the antiemetic domperidone.

> Apomorphine is ineffective orally but is a powerful dopaminergic D_1 and D_2 receptor agonist if given by subcutaneous or intramuscular injection. It can be an effective rescue treatment for rapidly occurring 'off' states or freezing. Apomorphine has also been developed as an intranasal or sublingual preparation, although this lengthens its time to take effect. This drug causes considerable nausea and vomiting and therefore domperidone therapy should be initiated prior to treatment. The major disadvantages of apomorphine therapy are its high cost (see Q. 5.12) and the requirements of a community support network to assist with the initiation and maintenance of therapy (see Q. 7.20).

7.18   How can apomorphine be used?

As a diagnostic test, as a rescue therapy or as a continuous infusion.

Apomorphine is frequently used to assess the possible response to treatment of a patient suspected to have Parkinson's disease – known as an apomorphine test (*see Q. 4.10*).

Some patients with advanced disease develop profound difficulties with treatment regimes and suffer from considerable disability as a result. Apomorphine can be used in these circumstances to 'rescue' a patient from severe parkinsonian symptoms until a more appropriate oral regime can be put in place. Where oral regimes fail to relieve parkinsonian symptoms without causing dyskinesias, apomorphine can be used as a continuous infusion to extend the duration of quality 'on' time.

7.19   How is apomorphine therapy introduced?

Test doses, and then can be used either intermittently or as a continuous infusion via a small subcutaneous needle.

Patients with advanced disease experiencing severely disabling fluctuations should be considered for apomorphine therapy. Patients require admission to hospital and at least 3 days' pretreatment with domperidone to minimise nausea and vomiting. Regular anti-parkinsonian medication should then be withheld overnight to render a patient in an 'off' state. The threshold of subcutaneous apomorphine necessary to restore function can then be assessed, and a patient (or carer) taught how to perform injections into the thighs or abdomen. Other anti-parkinsonian drugs can then be re-established. Patients requiring more than 10 injections per day may prefer a continuous infusion of apomorphine. Domperidone may normally be gradually withdrawn after several weeks.

7.20   What does a continuous infusion of apomorphine entail?

The infusion of apomorphine during the day via a small cannula in the abdominal wall and the involvement and support of specialist PD nurses and clinics.

In order for a patient to receive apomorphine infusions, an effective support network is essential. The majority of patients will require daily visits by a community nurse who has had experience in Parkinson's disease and the use of such infusions. The patient requires a supply of subcutaneous needles and syringes and a syringe driver pump (*Fig. 7.2*) which can be programmed to infuse the required dose of apomorphine over 18 hours. If patients can be stabilised on this treatment, it can lead to greatly improved control of 'on/off' fluctuations, over a period of time, similar to that seen with some surgical procedures (*see Ch. 8*).

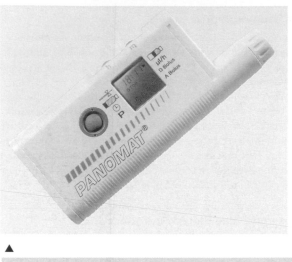

▲

Fig 7.2 An apomorphine infusion pump. Reproduced with permission of Disetronic Medical Systems AG.

7.21 Is there a maximum dose of L-dopa?

No but it is rare for patients to be on more than 1000–2000 mg per day.

In patients who show an initial response to small doses of L-dopa as monotherapy, the dose may need to be increased to as high as 1000 mg per day to provide symptom relief as the disease progresses. If greater relief is required, a dopamine agonist should then be given. In the days before dopamine agonists, patients were treated with 2000–3000 mg of L-dopa daily, but this tends to result in severe disabling dyskinesias.

In patients who show little or no response to L-dopa, a reasonably high dose before concluding that L-dopa is ineffective is 2000 mg per day. This can be an important piece of information in differentiating between Parkinson's disease and Parkinson-plus syndromes.

7.22 Does tolerance to L-dopa occur?

No.

Studies which have used continuous day and night intravenous or intraduodenal infusions of L-dopa have been found to elevate the threshold required to produce symptom relief, but daytime-only infusions actually reduced the requirement for the drug. It is therefore likely that increasing requirements of L-dopa by patients are due to disease progression rather than tolerance of the drug.

7.23   Is L-dopa addictive?

Not to any significant extent.

Many patients are *dependent* on L-dopa in order to maintain mobility and quality of life. This is not generally regarded as addiction. There have, however, been reports of Parkinson's disease patients rendered completely quadriplegic through other illnesses, who still demand L-dopa to prevent withdrawal symptoms such as anxiety, palpitations and sweating. It is known that elevated dopamine levels are involved in mechanisms of addiction to other drugs, suggesting that it may indeed be theoretically possible to become addicted to L-dopa itself. This remains speculative, though, with respect to PD and so should not in any way discourage prescription of the drug, given the enormous beneficial effects observed.

7.24   How can patients be treated who cannot swallow tablets?

Use dispersible forms of Madopar or apomorphine injections.

An intravenous form of L-dopa does exist but is only of value for research purposes. For patients who are unable to take oral forms of L-dopa, a dispersible form of Madopar exists that can be absorbed sublingually, or, alternatively, subcutaneous injections or infusions of apomorphine can be used. This may be sufficient to then allow patients to swallow their tablets normally.

Patients who are likely to be unable to swallow over long-term periods may also be treated with intraduodenal infusions of L-dopa plus decarboxylase inhibitor through percutaneous feeding tubes. This form of therapy is, however, not straightforward and requires the availability of an appropriate support infrastructure, only available through a few specialist centres. There are currently no rectal preparations of L-dopa.

7.25   How do I assess the patient with advanced Parkinson's disease?

 Establish timing of fluctuations, dyskinesias and nocturnal problems.

In order to evaluate the disability experienced by a patient with advanced Parkinson's disease and the effects of changing treatment regimes, it is important to ascertain:
- time spent 'on/off'
- best time of day
- worst time of day
- nocturnal symptoms
- occurrence of dyskinesias relative to medication timing.

Further adjustments of medication to minimise both PD symptoms and side-effects of medication can then be made.

7.26 Should all patients with advanced Parkinson's disease be attending specialist clinics?

Yes.

Patients with advanced Parkinson's disease require specialist knowledge to interpret the complicated symptoms that may be related to either deteriorating disease or side-effects from treatment.

PQ PATIENT QUESTIONS

Can the drug ecstasy stop dyskinesias?

Many people saw the television programme that featured a patient with young-onset Parkinson's disease, suffering from severe L-dopa-induced dyskinesias following many years of L-dopa treatment. This man had experimented with the drug ecstasy while dancing at a nightclub and had noticed a beneficial response in terms of his dyskinesias. The programme showed quite convincing evidence of an improvement in his dyskinesias following ecstasy intake.

There is ongoing research into the role of drugs like ecstasy as a way of treating drug-induced dyskinesias. Hopefully, this work will lead to the production of drugs that can be taken by patients who suffer from dyskinesias, without the side-effects of overexcitement and overheating that can dangerously complicate ecstasy intake and can even kill people. Such new drugs might benefit Parkinson's disease patients with advanced disease of all ages. At present, ecstasy is illegal, has dangerous side-effects, and cannot be recommended for patients with Parkinson's disease.

Could my dyskinesias have been avoided?

Dyskinesias are a common problem for people who have been treated for Parkinson's disease for more than 5 years, and they occur as a complication of all the drugs that work on the dopamine receptors. The knowledge that dyskinesias occur less frequently with the newer dopamine agonist drugs than with L-dopa has only been learned over the past 4–5 years, and this is the reason that more of the dopamine agonist type of drugs are now prescribed. L-dopa is still, however, the most effective drug for the relief of symptoms of Parkinson's disease. Unfortunately, even if treatment is started with a dopamine agonist drug rather than L-dopa, dyskinesias may still develop. The priority once this has happened should be to fine tune your treatment and so minimise the amount of dyskinesia periods you have to suffer from, without leaving you with too many symptoms of Parkinson's disease. In addition to changing the dose schedule for your L-dopa, a number of other drugs that have been shown to be useful in the treatment of dyskinesias can be tried. The one that should be tried first is called amantadine.

Why do my tablets not work on all occasions?

After you take one of your tablets, you may notice that your symptoms of Parkinson's disease start to improve after half an hour or so. The delay is due to the time it takes for the drug to get from your stomach into your bloodstream and then into the brain. Once enough of the drug has got to the right part of the brain, then the symptoms improve. Sometimes you may notice that you get very little improvement in your symptoms even after taking your normal dose of L-dopa. Various factors can slow down the uptake of drug between the stomach and the brain and sometimes the L-dopa never gets to the brain in high enough quantities to 'switch you on'. You might try taking your tablets a short time before meals to see if this helps. Another option is to take either a slow-release form of L-dopa or a drug called entacapone, which stops the L-dopa being broken down in the bloodstream, so that more L-dopa can get into your brain and 'switch you on'.

Is my Parkinson's disease ever going to be controlled again?

The swings between the symptoms of Parkinson's disease and terrible dyskinetic movements can cause considerable difficulties. When almost all of the tablet combinations have been tried and none has achieved acceptable symptom control, the next step is to try a drug called apomorphine, which has to be given by injection. You will need to be admitted to hospital to start this medication and be taught how to inject yourself. Surgery too is a possibility, and it may be appropriate to refer you to a surgeon with experience of the new surgical procedures for Parkinson's disease, who may be able to help you.

Surgical treatments for Parkinson's disease

8

8.1 What surgical procedures have been used in Parkinson's disease?

Lesioning or deep brain stimulation of critical regions of the brain called the thalamus, globus pallidus, and subthalamic nucleus.

There have been three general approaches to treating Parkinson's disease surgically (*Fig. 8.1*).

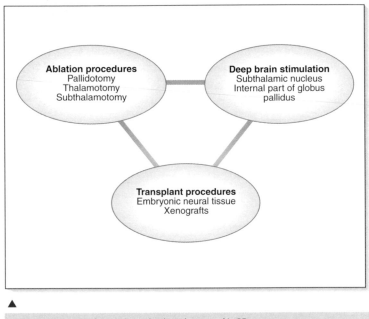

▲

Fig. 8.1 The surgical procedures that have been used in PD.

The original surgical methods involved performing an ablation procedure to lesion various parts of the basal ganglia, namely the thalamus, subthalamus, and globus pallidus; giving rise to the terms thalamotomy, subthalamotomy, and pallidotomy.

More recently, stimulating electrodes have been placed within similar deep regions of the basal ganglia, and the patients fitted with a power supply to stimulate their brains. This procedure is known as deep brain stimulation.

Various groups have attempted or are currently attempting to transplant cells into the basal ganglia that might grow and make connections with the host cells and subsequently restore normal dopamine production, and so cure patients of PD.

8.2 Which patients should be considered for surgery?

Motivated, non-demented patients with advanced poorly controlled disease.

At present, medical therapy is usually able to effectively relieve the symptoms of Parkinson's disease for about 5–10 years following diagnosis. The discovery of new drugs for PD is extending this period during which good medical control of symptoms is possible. As the disease progresses, the quality of life of some patients deteriorates because of prolonged 'off' periods and intolerable dyskinesias during 'on' periods. Patients suffering from such severe disability but still showing a transient beneficial response from L-dopa should be considered for functional neurosurgery procedures. Such patients should be in otherwise good general health without dementia or severe depression and with normal brain imaging.

8.3 What is a pallidotomy?

A procedure that lesions a part of the basal ganglia called the globus pallidus (*see Table 8.1*).

Loss of dopamine within the substantia nigra leads to increased activity in the internal part of the globus pallidus (GPi). This nucleus has inhibitory effects over the thalamus, cortex and brainstem, which lead to the bradykinesia seen in Parkinson's disease patients (*Fig. 8.2*). L-dopa therapy initially restores the excessive inhibitory effects of the GPi; however, chronic dopamine replacement therapy leads to the development of drug-induced dyskinesias (*see Q. 7.12*). Surgical ablation of a part of the globus pallidus – a pallidotomy – has been shown to primarily reduce the severity of drug-induced dyskinesias and dystonia on the contralateral side without dramatically changing the underlying features of the PD. In some patients who are not able to tolerate medical treatment owing to the severity of their dyskinesias, pallidotomy surgery can help allow patients to get back onto effective treatment. However, given its modest effects on the underlying PD, the procedure is now becoming superseded by other surgical procedures.

8.4 What is the role for thalamotomy?

An old-fashioned procedure that primarily helps patients with severe tremor (*see Table 8.1*).

Prior to the discovery of L-dopa, it was observed that tremor can be helped by lesioning the contralateral ventral intermediate nucleus (VIM nucleus) of the thalamus, a procedure termed 'a thalamotomy'. Targeting the ventrolateral thalamus can also improve rigidity, but may worsen bradykinesia and gait difficulties. Thalamotomy is now rarely done (less than 5% of surgical procedures for Parkinson's disease), and is reserved for

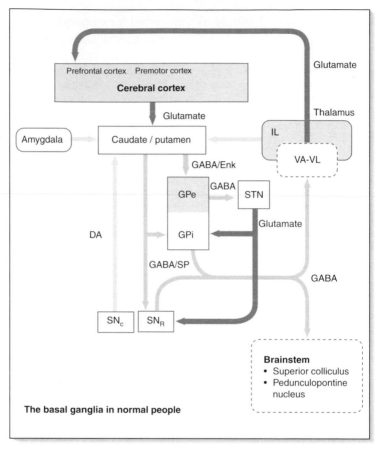

A

Fig. 8.2 Schematic figure of basal ganglia and flow charts of activity changes in health and disease. DA, dopamine; Enk, enkephalin; GABA, γ-aminobutyric acid; GPe, globus pallidus – external segment; GPi, globus pallidus – internal segment; IL, intralaminar nuclei of thalamus; SN$_C$, substantia nigra pars compacta; SN$_R$, substantia nigra pars reticulata; SP, substance P; STN, subthalamic nucleus; VA-VL, ventroanterior-ventrolateral nuclei of thalamus.

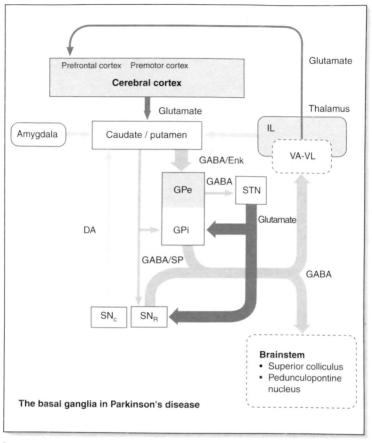

Fig. 8.2 (*Cont'd*) Schematic figure of basal ganglia and flow charts of activity changes in health and disease. DA, dopamine; Enk, enkephalin; GABA, γ-aminobutyric acid; GPe, globus pallidus – external segment; GPi, globus pallidus – internal segment; IL, intralaminar nuclei of thalamus; SN_C, substantia nigra pars compacta; SN_R, substantia nigra pars reticulata; SP, substance P; STN, subthalamic nucleus; VA-VL, ventroanterior-ventrolateral nuclei of thalamus.

TABLE 8.1 Lesion procedures performed for PD patients

	Pallidotomy	Thalamotomy	Subthalamotomy
Target	Internal part of globus pallidus (GPi)	VIM nucleus of the thalamus	Subthalamic nucleus
Symptomatic indication	Drug treatments causing uncontrollable dyskinesia and dystonia	Intractable tremor	Severe PD symptoms uncontrolled by medication
Mechanism of symptom improvement	Prevents inhibitory output of the GPi	Unclear	Prevents STN excitation of the GPi

patients with severe disabling tremor. Bilateral thalamotomy is associated with significant morbidity and is not recommended.

8.5 What is a subthalamotomy?

A lesion of another part of the basal ganglia called the subthalamic nucleus (*see Table 8.1*).

The subthalamic nucleus (STN) has an excitatory effect on the GPi, and therefore this nucleus has been considered as an alternative target to alleviate the PD symptoms attributable to an overactive GPi. Patients have therefore been treated by subthalamotomy with some encouraging results, although the efficacy and safety of this procedure remain controversial. Ablation of the subthalamic nucleus can produce marked contralateral improvement in akinesia, rigidity and tremor, but there is a small risk of ballismus (defined as large flailing limb movements). Subthalamotomies do not appear to have any beneficial effects on dyskinesias. There is less experience with this procedure than with pallidotomy, and most experts would now recommend deep brain stimulation (*see Q. 8.8*) over lesion surgery, if this is available.

8.6 How is a surgical lesion made?

By insertion of a small electrode, through which a small accurately placed lesion is made.

Surgical lesions are made by electrocoagulation of the target through a fine needle. The needle needs extremely accurate placement within the brain to avoid damaging vital structures. This is achieved through MRI imaging prior to surgery and the use of a stereotactic frame to guarantee that the needle is placed into precise coordinates. Whilst surgery can be done under a general anaesthetic, many centres prefer to have the patient awake so that the effects of the procedure can be monitored by passing small non-lesioning electrical impulses down the electrode. This reduces the

Most of the pioneering work of DBS has been performed outside of the UK, especially in France. The procedure is currently being further evaluated in a trial in the UK in order to assess its effects on the quality of life and its cost-effectiveness. At the present time, however, the procedure is still not widely available, and so, whilst the results of the few centres that have experience of the procedure are promising, the vast majority of patients will not currently have access to this procedure.

In areas where the procedure is being performed, patients are being selected on the basis of who is most likely to benefit. Currently, the procedure is being reserved for patients who are relatively young, still have some response to a dose of L-dopa, and are free from significant dementia.

8.11 Can patients stop medical treatment after successful surgery?

Yes, although in most cases patients still require some medical therapy.

The benefits of surgical treatments on some of the symptoms of Parkinson's disease may be obvious immediately following the surgery. Some patients show such benefits that greatly reduced amounts of dopaminergic therapy are needed. However, most patients still require some medication, and in certain procedures such as pallidotomy, the procedure may actually allow a patient to go back onto treatment, as dyskinesias are less of a problem.

8.12 Do surgical treatments for Parkinson's disease improve all the features of it?

Probably not.

Of the various studies looking at cognitive impairments in Parkinson's disease patients before and after surgery (be it pallidotomy or deep brain stimulation), most (but not all) have shown a slight deterioration. This is in obvious contrast to the large benefits in motor symptoms that can be seen after such treatments. Recent work suggests that there may be small benefits on subtle testing, but that this is very much related to the exact anatomical site targeted by the procedure. It is felt that this may be a limiting factor in the widespread adoption of this procedure.

8.13 Can transplant surgery help in Parkinson's disease?

Probably, but it remains an unproven, experimental therapy.

Attempts have been made to implant tissue capable of producing dopamine into the brains of patients with advanced Parkinson's disease. The initial work used tissue transplanted from the patient's own adrenal gland into the striatum. Initial encouraging responses were disappointingly followed by a return to the pre-transplant parkinsonian state, and post-mortem reports have confirmed that these transplanted cells do not survive.

Concentration has now focused on the possible transplantation of human embryonic tissue into the brains of PD patients. Such transplants have been performed with a variable range of results, and there has been some concern that a small percentage of patients receiving transplants may have worsening of their dyskinesias following the procedure. It is likely, however, that improvement in techniques will confirm the usefulness of this procedure in carefully selected patients. This is currently an experimental procedure, which is being evaluated in a few centres, and is not available for patients with PD in the UK.

Transplantation of tissue from other species such as pig, has also been considered for patients with PD, but there are major problems with such an approach and it remains a long way off from the clinic. Patients can obtain transplants of this and similar animals through a number of web-based sites, but such approaches are unproven, unethical and dangerous.

8.14 What is stem cell therapy?

Stem cells are a type of cell that can divide and give rise to new cells, including those of the brain.

Neural stem cells are cells that are capable of both proliferation and differentiation into the main types of brain cells. Stem cells can be found in both the adult and embryonic brain, and cells from these sources can be harvested and grown in the laboratory. Whilst there is a great deal of research investigating the use of these cells for transplantation in Parkinson's disease, the work is not yet advanced enough for evaluation of efficacy within human subjects. The various types of stem cell therapy are described in Table 8.2.

8.15 What are xenografts?

Transplants of tissue from one species (e.g. pig) to another (e.g. human).

Xenografts are cells that are harvested from the tissues of one species and transplanted into another species. Xenografts have been considered for several years as a source of organs for both heart, and liver transplants, and research is in progress regarding the possibility of using animal tissue as a source of dopamine-producing cells that might be transplanted into the

TABLE 8.2 Stem cell types being considered for transplantation in PD

Cell type	Source	Disadvantages
Adult neural stem cell	Adult brain	No ethical problems with obtaining cells, but difficulties in deriving and growing sufficient numbers of such cells
Embryonic stem (ES) cell	In vitro fertilisation (IVF) clinics	Substantial ethical concerns, and difficulty in getting cells to grow only into nerve cells and not a host of different types of cells
Embryonic neural stem cell	Human fetuses aborted for other reasons, then grown in culture in the laboratory	Ethical concerns persist. Difficulty with getting cells to turn into dopamine nerve cells
Xenograft	Specially reared pig embryos	Ethical concerns, risk of transmission of infection from pig to human and rejection of tissue by immune system as it is recognised as being foreign by human immune system

brains of Parkinson's disease sufferers. The species that is being most closely considered for this role are pigs. This is because their brains are approximately the same physical size as humans, and therefore they have cells which grow to the same approximate size as human cells. Pig tissues also share many important features in common with humans and are easily bred, and thus would represent a ready supply of embryonic brain tissue.

The main disadvantages arising in the field of xenotransplantation are in terms of preventing rejection and minimising risk of cross-species transmission of infection. There are also ethical concerns with raising animals solely for human therapies.

8.16 Was transplant therapy not shown recently to have catastrophic results?

Yes, but there were major problems with this trial.

An American team performed a randomised controlled trial of the effects of transplanting human fetal tissue into the brains of patients with advanced PD. One group of patients received the fetal tissue injected into the striatum, and another group went to the operating theatre, were anaesthetised but had only burr-holes drilled into the skull. In this way, patients were unaware whether they had received a transplant or not.

All the patients were followed up for at least 1 year. An improvement in patient symptoms was noticed in the majority of young-onset patients who had received transplants, in comparison with the control group. For this reason, many of the control group patients also went on to receive transplanted tissue themselves. Further follow-up discovered that 17% of the treated patients had developed dyskinesias after 2–3 years without taking any L-dopa treatment. This adverse aspect to the treatment caused much publicity in the international press, with little attention directed towards the benefits seen in many of the patients.

Other groups that are involved in transplant therapies have criticised the techniques used in this study, and argue that more fundamental research should have been done. This study is therefore far from conclusive but does highlight the dangers and experimental nature of this procedure.

PQ PATIENT QUESTIONS

Can I not have an operation for my Parkinson's disease?

You are quite right that there are operations that exist that can be very useful for Parkinson's disease patients. Some of these operations involve destroying tiny parts of the brain, and have been performed for many years for patients with very severe tremor, or in very severe cases where drugs are causing uncontrollable involuntary movements called dyskinesias. There are also new types of operations that use deep brain stimulators to excite bits of the brain, and these are being used for people who have severe symptoms of Parkinson's disease that cannot be controlled with tablets.

Whilst such operations can be very successful, an operation is not advised at a stage when tablets are able to control your symptoms. Even though they are becoming increasingly safe procedures, there are still significant risks associated with these operations, such as strokes, blindness or even death. Also, at the moment, they are only available in a very few places, though it is hoped that there will be more surgeons able to perform them over the next few years.

Is it true that the brains of unborn babies are being used for Parkinson's disease?

There is research that involves the use of cells from human embryos as possible treatments for Parkinson's disease. This type of research is controversial and raises a number of ethical issues. If a woman in the early stages of pregnancy wants to have an abortion in the UK, she is able to ask for this to be done within the National Health Service. After the procedure, the tissue from the aborted embryo is usually incinerated.

In certain parts of the country, women who have decided to have an abortion are told about the research into brain diseases such as Parkinson's disease, and asked if they would give their permission for a few cells from the embryonic tissue to be used as part of this research. This is rigorously regulated and strict guidelines exist for the use of such tissue. However, some of this tissue has been used in patients with Parkinson's disease, with some encouraging results. This procedure is still an experimental one and as such is not available.

Non-drug treatment of Parkinson's disease, and social issues

9

PQ PATIENT QUESTIONS

9.1 What are non-drug treatments and what aspects of Parkinson's disease can be helped by them?

Education, support and advice can help all aspects of PD in part.

There are many issues that confront a patient who has developed Parkinson's disease, and of these, many can be assisted by non-drug interventions as well as drug treatment. The consultation between doctor and patient should therefore be an important time to identify which day-to-day problems are most disabling to an individual patient, and have not been adequately relieved by drug therapy. Physicians should consider themselves as a source of education, support, and advice for PD patients regarding their disease, as well as providing and monitoring the effects of drug therapy. In addition, patients may derive great benefit and information by contacting their local PD society branch through the national office (see Q. 11.5).

Simple matters such as exercise and nutrition, writing, cooking, washing, dressing, driving a car, sexual dysfunction and a patient's ability to interact socially are often neglected, as motor disabilities and drug regimes dominate the consultation. Identifying how PD affects a patient's quality of life is now recognised as a particularly important part of patient care. It is very important to remember the huge benefit that occupational therapy, physiotherapy, and speech therapy can offer for PD patients.

9.2 How do we assess a Parkinson's disease patient's quality of life?

PD-specific rating scales exist.

There are numerous reasons for the decrease in quality of life suffered by Parkinson's disease patients: loss of mobility, falls, depression, social embarrassment, isolation, sleep disturbances, dyskinesias and fluctuations. In a routine consultation attention may not be paid to these aspects of PD that significantly impact on the patient's quality of life. There are now several useful measures of quality of life that have been designed for patients with PD, and have been validated in large-scale studies, which can act as a checklist during a consultation. The most reliable of these is the PDQ-39 which directs questions at 39 different quality of life aspects that are most commonly impaired by PD. These 39 questions focus on the following eight categories and the results are presented as eight discrete scores:

1. Mobility (e.g. fear of falling when walking)
2. Activities of daily living (e.g. difficulty cutting food)
3. Emotional well-being (e.g. feelings of isolation)
4. Stigma (e.g. social embarrassment)
5. Social support

6. Cognition
7. Communication
8. Bodily discomfort.

Higher scores are consistently associated with the more severe symptoms of the disease such as tremor and stiffness. A copy of the PDQ-39 is reproduced in Appendix 1.

9.3 What simple advice can help patients with Parkinson's disease?

Adaptation of many simple household implements and routines can be of great benefit.

Many everyday activities can be made more simple for Parkinson's disease patients by planning and modifying existing household items, and appropriate discussion can identify many possible ways to do this. Writing can be made easier by using a different style of pen, or by using an alternative such as a typewriter, computer or audio tape to replace the need for pens and paper altogether. Meals should be planned to avoid foods that require complicated preparation, or foods that are tough and therefore difficult to cut. If lifting dishes out of a low oven is difficult, a microwave or other methods of cooking could be used.

Special utensils, lightweight pans, large-handled cutlery, or even straws can make cooking, eating and drinking a less arduous task.

Poor dexterity which impairs dressing abilities can be less of a disability if items such as slip-on shoes, clip-on ties, or Velcro fasteners are used. Bathroom modifications can help to ensure safety and optimise independence, especially the use of electric toothbrushes or razors to replace traditional items. Turning over in bed may be made simpler by the use of lightweight duvets or satin sheets rather than heavy blankets.

A patient's domestic function may be best observed at first hand as part of an occupational therapy assessment.

9.4 How can occupational therapy help in Parkinson's disease?

By assessing patients in their own homes and making the necessary modifications.

Occupational therapists (OTs) can provide invaluable assessments to optimise a patient's environment in the home and in some cases also the workplace. This can be most useful in the early stages of the disease to prevent problems from developing. The OT can evaluate a patient getting in and out of bed, eating, dressing, and bathing and advise and recommend simple techniques to optimise activities of daily living and create an environment which minimises the risk of falls. The therapist can also advise on the training and use of specialist adaptive household equipment or provide simple advice such as replacing a bath with a shower.

The OT's involvement may also include finding and completing application forms for special equipment and advising on sources of funding for often-expensive adaptive aids. Occupational therapists can be found through either hospital or community health services or through the address below:

The College of Occupational Therapists
6–8 Marshalsea Road
Southwark
London
SE1 1HL
www.cot.org.uk

9.5 Is there a role for physiotherapy?

Yes, especially with respect to gait and mobility.

Physiotherapy is invaluable for Parkinson's disease patients as a source of advice on, and treatment of, mobility problems including posture, turning and freezing. Early referral is useful so that both the patient and the caregiver can be taught techniques to keep joints mobile, perform muscle stretches, and maintain strength. The physiotherapist can also make an assessment of balance problems that cause falling and advise on the use of crutches, canes or walking frames. Local physiotherapists can be found through either hospital or community health services, or through the following address:

Chartered Society for Physiotherapists
14 Bedford Row
London
WC1R 4ED
www.csphysio.org.uk

Physiotherapists may also teach group sessions as part of Parkinson's Disease Society meetings.

9.6 How can patients improve their gait?

By attending to correct posture and concentrating on their walking.

Emphasis on correct posture and relearning patterns of walking are an important part of preventing falls and maintaining mobility. Patients should be reminded to stand up straight, lengthen their stride and lift their feet during walking. Sensible non-slip shoes should be worn, potential hazards should be removed and handrails should be recommended for patients with significant postural instability. These suggestions and recommendations can often best be made by the physiotherapists and OTs.

As the disease advances, patients may need to be taught how to turn around safely using a short-stepped U-turn rather than pivoting on the spot. Patients can be trained to consciously centre their feet under their body and thus to provide themselves with a more stable platform and so minimise the risk of falling, particularly when arising from a chair.

9.7 What physical tricks help overcome freezing?

A number exist which rely on sensory cues to trick the brain into initiating a movement.

Freezing episodes are a frequent complication of PD and commonly occur when a patient is confronted by a narrow doorway or tight space. There are several non-pharmacological tricks which can improve mobility when it is compromised by freezing episodes. Patients can be taught to look through a doorway to a target in the next room, or may be helped by counting during walking, the natural rhythm of which often allows the patient to walk for longer distances. (Counting, however, can sometimes impair a patient's concentration and as a result a patient may be more prone to falling. All advice should therefore be tailored according to a patient's response and capabilities.)

Many patients have benefited from having strips of tape stuck to their carpets or floors, which they have to step over and by so doing can help prevent freezing from occurring. Indeed, many patients may be able to overcome an episode of freezing simply by imagining that they are stepping over a low obstacle in front of them. Alternatively, the carer can help by

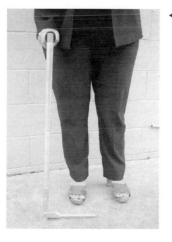

Fig. 9.1 The Kickstart Stick (courtesy of John Green). Further information can be obtained from Dr John Green, 1 Tofanella Street, Fig Tree Pocket, Queensland, Australia 4069; email: kickstart@qldnet.au.

providing such cues. Various specially developed walking sticks are available that have been modified to help provide a stimulus that a patient can step over in order to overcome freezing episodes. Such modifications include either a short horizontal bar jutting out from the bottom end of the stick (*Fig. 9.1*), or a stick that can shine a beam of light across the floor in front of the patient. Both of these provide a non-hazardous stimulus that the patient can use to 'step over' and overcome the freezing attack.

9.8 How much physical exercise should be recommended?

No absolute amount can be stipulated, but regular exercise is important.

Parkinson's disease patients need specific advice on exercise programmes in order to maintain muscle strength and flexibility, and prevent disuse atrophy of muscles. In addition to locomotor and cardiovascular benefits, exercise is also useful to enhance mood and diminish stress as well as help with constipation. Patients should be advised to exercise at a time when their medication is optimal, and the type of exercise routine and duration should be realistically tailored to each patient. Non-weightbearing exercise such as swimming or aqua-aerobics may be particularly suited to PD patients (provided adequate supervision exists), and patients should be advised to avoid sports that might be dangerous should a freezing episode occur. There is no upper limit of exercise for patients with high levels of fitness, although patients should not exercise to the point of exhaustion. There is no evidence that physical exercise retards or accelerates the disease process.

9.9 How can speech be improved?

Speech therapy involvement is often helpful in patients with PD, many of whom have difficulties with their speech volume and articulation.

Slurred, quiet, or dysarthric speech can be a particularly frustrating symptom of Parkinson's disease. Patients are able to raise their voices if given a cue such as when speaking to someone in another room, but often are unable to gauge the appropriate volume at which to speak when talking face to face. The patient should be instructed to deliberately speak louder, always look directly at the person with whom they are talking, exaggerate their pronunciation, use shorter sentences and consciously breathe between sentences. Patient should be encouraged to use their voice frequently, and not allow others to finish their sentences for them. Speech therapy can often be helpful, especially if the patient is also experiencing swallowing difficulties.

9.10 Is there anything that helps with swallowing?

Dopaminergic therapies are often helpful for PD patients with swallowing difficulties.

Swallowing can be a neglected problem for many Parkinson's disease patients. Patients often need to consciously think about their swallowing to compensate for loss of the swallow reflex. Taking smaller bites of food and alternating food with sips of drink can be helpful. Early referral to a speech and language therapist may ensure optimal swallowing instruction and advice regarding choice of food types. In some cases, there is a problem of aspiration of food particles or liquids and this can lead to breathing difficulties and recurrent pneumonia. In such circumstances, urgent referral to a speech therapist is needed with a view to videofluoroscopy of swallowing to identify the nature, and extent, of aspiration and risk of continued oral intake of food and drink. If this reveals significant problems or there are severe difficulties with swallowing, then the patient may require treatment with percutaneous gastrostomy and/or alternative methods of administering medication (*see Q. 7.20*).

Finally, it is important to be certain that swallowing difficulties are attributable to PD rather than other causes such as an oesophageal pouch or carcinoma. Speech therapy assessment with videofluoroscopy can also help to resolve this issue.

9.11   Are any dietary modifications useful?

Usually not, although some patients benefit from a protein redistribution diet.

It is important to monitor a patient's weight from one consultation to the next, especially in patients with advanced disease. Although some Parkinson's disease patients put on weight because of loss of mobility and subsequent inactivity, the majority of patients lose weight because of insufficient calorie intake, swallowing difficulties or inability to prepare meals. Dyskinetic patients also use large quantities of energy during their dyskinesias which can contribute further to weight loss.

All patients should be informed about what constitutes a balanced diet, with emphasis placed on fibre and plenty of fluid intake, both of which can help to prevent constipation. Osteoporosis is also common among the PD population and the PD patient is more likely to suffer fractures of the hip or other bones, since the risk for falling is higher with parkinsonian symptoms. Therefore the patient should be advised on foods rich in calcium, and be prescribed vitamin D or bisphosphonates if evidence of osteoporosis exists.

Motor fluctuations (*see Q. 7.3*) may be influenced by the amount of protein eaten. Protein is broken down into amino acids during digestion, which compete with L-dopa for absorption from the intestine. The more protein which is ingested, the longer the L-dopa may take to work (owing to its reduced uptake), the less effective it may be and the sooner it may wear off. Consideration is therefore given in some patients to shift their protein intake toward the evening or, alternatively, they should try to schedule protein-containing meals in the middle of dose intervals. Carbohydrates enhance L-dopa absorption into the brain by removing competing amino acids, and can further improve patients suffering from unpredictable fluctuations.

Patients with persistent weight loss may benefit from referral to a dietician. When difficulty with cooking is the main problem, assistance from support services such as 'Meals on Wheels' may be necessary. Patients with significant swallowing difficulties may be appropriate for percutaneous feeding through a PEG tube (*see Qs 2.21 and 7.20*).

9.12 What is the role of Parkinson's disease specialist nurses?

To support, educate and advise patient, carer, family and GP.

There are a growing number of Parkinson's disease specialist nurses (PDSNs) working throughout the UK. These nurses have a wealth of experience of PD, and are often the main source of support, counselling and education for a patient. As well as providing education for patients regarding their disease, PDSNs are more able to visit patients at home, can coordinate care packages and input from social services and offer specialist advice for both patients and carers. Minor alterations in drug dosing and drug timing can be advised by the PDSN in response to changes in drug requirements or side-effects and this can help reduce the burden on the general practitioner. PDSNs are invaluable in supervising patients through complex medication changes and particularly when apomorphine therapy is required.

The PDSN also fills a vital role liaising between consultant specialist, GPs, the PD Society and other health professionals and thus provides a multidisciplinary approach to the management of patient care.

9.13 Can anything help with sexual dysfunction in Parkinson's disease?

Yes, advice and modification of therapy with consideration of using sildenafil (Viagra).

Parkinson's patients often have impaired sexual function for a variety of reasons. Loss of agility and flexibility may make it physically very difficult to perform sexually, which may be improved with optimising anti-PD medication. Depression and anxiety are not uncommon as reasons for loss of interest in sexual intercourse, and appropriate treatment should again be considered. Some of the drugs used to treat PD (including β-blockers) may also have side-effects that reduce libido or sexual potency. Other drugs that can induce impotence include α-adrenergic blockers, thiazide diuretics, anxiolytics, digoxin, cimetidine, and some antidepressants.

Loss of female libido may respond to subcutaneous testosterone implants, and lubricant creams should be prescribed as necessary. Medical evaluation of sexual dysfunction in male and female patients can be determined by obtaining serum levels of prolactin, testosterone, luteinising hormone, and thyroid function studies, and appropriate referral can be made if necessary. Drugs such as sildenafil (Viagra) may have a role but it is also important to ensure that couples are also able to plan time for intimacy.

Hypersexuality is not uncommon with dopaminergic drugs, and occasionally requires medication change, for instance a change from one dopamine agonist to another.

9.14 Is there any benefit to be had in taking homeopathic medicines for Parkinson's disease?

It is unknown whether such therapies help.

Many Parkinson's disease patients consult homeopathy practitioners who prescribe treatments for 'individuals' rather than for 'diseases', and many patients feel that they benefit from such consultations. There may be a significant placebo effect involved in observed benefits but it may be that the placebo effect is mediated through increased release of dopamine as has been shown in healthy volunteers using PET scans.

Patients should, however, be warned that homeopathic remedies are often not cheap. If benefit is obtained from homeopathic medications, there is usually little to be gained in trying to persuade a patient to stop these treatments, unless there is an obvious contraindication, e.g. pregnancy.

An ancient Indian medical remedy for PD uses '*Mucuna pruriens*' as a treatment for the disease. A study from the United States reports this to be a safe and effective treatment, although more must be learned about it before we conclude that this offers more than a placebo effect. Additionally, fava beans have been found to contain naturally occurring L-dopa in high levels and can be taken as a 'natural' remedy, in soups or purées. However, people with a hereditary condition commonly known as favism must not eat these beans.

9.15 Are other complementary therapies useful?

Probably, although their mode of action is often not clear.

 In addition to traditional medical services, a variety of complementary therapies may enhance the physical and emotional well-being of a Parkinson's disease patient. Massage therapy may promote relaxation and may reduce the symptoms of tremor and rigidity. Controlled breathing exercises and yoga are also found to be beneficial by some patients.

There is little evidence available from randomised trials regarding these and other therapies such as aromatherapy or acupuncture. Of the little trial evidence available, acupuncture has been associated with an improved lifestyle and yoga, apart from causing a few aches and pains in the overenthusiastic, also proved very beneficial. Hypnotherapy may provide an improvement in relaxation, although reflexology has not produced any positive results from the limited data that are available. Patients who find these alternative therapies useful, and are not suffering any detrimental side-effects, should not be discouraged from pursuing these treatments. Surveys of the use of complementary therapies in PD suggest that the majority of patients who use them are from higher social classes, which is likely to be due to the substantial expense of these treatments.

9.16 Can patients drive with Parkinson's disease?

Yes, assuming they are not severely disabled by their PD, and do not have sleep attacks due to their treatment.

Many patients with Parkinson's disease are significantly concerned about the consequences that the diagnosis may have on their legal status with respect to driving. Patients with PD may have no difficulties at all with driving, and can perfectly safely remain behind the wheel. However, a range of difficulties with driving may be experienced by patients with established disease, including those with severe movement problems that are not controlled, unpredictable motor fluctuations, drug-induced drowsiness, or cognitive deficits. In such circumstances, the patient should not drive. Patients with more minor disabilities who are safe to drive may benefit from power steering or driving cars with automatic gearboxes. Sophisticated vehicle adaptation is also now possible and includes joysticks and infrared controls for people who are severely disabled.

The DVLA in Swansea will need to know which, if any, of the controls require to be modified and will ask the patient to complete a simple questionnaire. The driving licence will then be coded to reflect the modifications.

9.17 Should the DVLA be informed about the diagnosis?

Yes.

Full details on the laws for driving within the UK can be found on the DVLA's web site:
www.dvla.gov.uk

A patient is legally obliged to inform the DVLA about any medical diagnoses that *may* cause disability, and this includes Parkinson's disease. The address for contacting the DVLA is:

Drivers Medical Unit
DVLA
Swansea
SA99 1TU

Contacting the DVLA does not necessarily imply that a patient will be stopped from driving. This depends on the level of disability experienced by an individual patient. The DVLA will write to the patient with a medical questionnaire which also asks for permission to approach the general practitioner and/or hospital consultant about the fitness of an individual with PD to drive. If there is doubt, then an independent assessment and/or driving test may be arranged by the DVLA.

Responsibility for taxi licensing rests entirely with the Public Carriage Office in the metropolitan area and with the local authority in the rest of the country. The various licensing authorities determine the standards to be applied for the issue of such licences in their area; this includes the determination of any medical standards.

The DVLA has no influence over, or involvement in, these procedures.

In patients with PD who have had surgical procedures such as pallidotomy or deep brain stimulation, the patient's licence must be revoked for 6 months, after which a further medical assessment must be made to ensure the patient is safe to restart driving.

9.18 Should a patient stop work following a diagnosis of Parkinson's disease?

No, unless it is impossible to continue despite adequate drug therapy.

Many patients are able to keep active working lives for many years after the onset of symptoms of Parkinson's disease. Where patients suffer from particular disabilities, they may benefit from identifying their particular responsibilities and tasks involved at work and finding ways of modifying their jobs to allow for this disability. When it becomes impossible to adequately modify the current role, and patients can envisage the job becoming 'at risk', they are best advised to seek alternative, physically less demanding roles within the same company or department rather than persisting at a task that is becoming more and more difficult.

Work-related stress should be minimised and patients should consider the best organisation of their time at work and ergonomically structure their environment. It is important to encourage people to continue working, as the disease runs a long course and premature retirement on health grounds can precipitate depression.

9.19 Should patients inform their employer about the diagnosis?

Not necessarily but it is often helpful if the employer is aware of the diagnosis. Patients with mild symptoms are under no obligation to inform their employer that they have Parkinson's disease. For patients with symptoms that are visible or obvious, it is often sensible to inform employers and colleagues about the diagnosis to avoid speculation and gossip. Often, greater support can be given by the employer following full discussion of the diagnosis, and appropriate modifications can then be made to the workplace to minimise the impact at work.

9.20 Can a patient be sacked for having Parkinson's disease?

No.

A patient cannot be sacked for having Parkinson's disease. An unreasonable employer who invents other reasons to dismiss someone with PD is acting illegally. Advice should be sought from trade unions or lawyers if patients feel that they have been unfairly dismissed.

9.21 How does a patient get disability benefits?

This is best arranged through the PD specialist nurse and the local social services department.

Patients are often unaware of their entitlements to disability benefits. Full information regarding entitlements and benefits is available through social services departments who can be contacted directly, or by visiting or phoning the local Citizens' Advice Bureau. Local information regarding day centres, luncheon clubs, respite care, night sitting services, home care, 'Meals on Wheels', home adaptations and residential care should also be available.

9.22 Can a patient get any compensation after developing Parkinson's disease?

Not usually, as the cause of PD remains unknown in most cases.

Many people are now protected by various insurance policies, or types of critical illness cover. Many of these policies will pay out lump sums following the diagnosis of Parkinson's disease. People worried that they might be at risk of developing chronic neurological diseases such as PD should be advised to buy cover from an insurance company that has been selling long-term care policies for at least 10 years and is financially sound with a high rating from insurance ratings services.

Patients who feel that they have developed their disease following exposure to chemicals or toxins at work may assume that they should be entitled to compensation through an industrial tribunal. The case for proving that industrial chemicals or environments were the cause for an individual's PD symptoms would be very difficult indeed to make.

PQ PATIENT QUESTIONS

I cannot get an erection. Could it be due to the Parkinson's disease?

Parkinson's disease is not generally the cause of difficulties getting or maintaining an erection, and when it is responsible, erections tend to improve again with the standard anti-PD drugs. Patients sometimes become more worried about sex because of the stress of the illness, or if the Parkinson's disease is stopping them moving around the bed. Problems with sex can also occur for reasons that have nothing to do with Parkinson's disease, and blood tests should be done to check on these before decisions are made about treatment.

What exercise can I do at my age?

Exercise is not only for the young and fit. You may find that taking regular exercise not only improves your mobility, but also improves your confidence and provides a useful outlet to interact with other people socially. Swimming might provide an excellent source of exercise for you, and so it is worth finding at what time the local pool runs sessions that suit you most. Once this is known, the timing of your medication can be adjusted to ensure that you can go along when you are at your most mobile.

Should I eat anything special to help my Parkinson's disease?

It is important that you continue with a balanced diet to keep you healthy, and you should continue to try to keep your weight stable. Plenty of fluids and fibre in the diet can prevent you from becoming constipated, but there are no foods that are *proven* to be beneficial for the symptoms of Parkinson's disease.

Differential diagnoses of Parkinson's disease and their relevance for the GP

10.1   What is parkinsonism?

The development of the clinical triad of rigidity, bradykinesia and tremor, for whatever reason.

'Parkinsonism' refers to the combination of slowness of movement, rigidity and tremor, which can be caused by any disease process affecting the basal ganglia, in particular the connections between the substantia nigra and the striatum. Many processes can lead to disruption or interruption of these connections, and the term 'Parkinson's disease' should be restricted to those patients with loss of this dopaminergic projection because of selective neurodegeneration for which no cause can clearly be identified. A large number of other processes can also disrupt these connections, including structural lesions and drugs that block the dopamine pathway. In addition there is a group of disorders in which there is degeneration of the nigrostriatal pathway as part of a more generalised neurodegenerative process. These other neurodegenerative processes are known as the Parkinson-plus diseases and are discussed further below (*see Q. 10.2*).

In practice it is often difficult to distinguish between Parkinson's disease and some of the other causes of parkinsonism. The causes of secondary parkinsonism and Parkinson-plus syndromes are summarised in Table 10.1.

TABLE 10.1   The causes of secondary parkinsonism and Parkinson-plus syndromes – the more important causes are highlighted in bold type

Causes of secondary parkinsonism	Examples
Infections	Post-encephalitis lethargica (extremely rare) Other viral encephalitides including Japanese B encephalitis, HIV (rare)
Toxins	Manganese, carbon monoxide, carbon disulphide, cyanide, methanol, MPTP (all rare)
Drugs	**Neuroleptics, dopamine antagonist antiemetics** (common) Reserpine, tetrabenazine, alpha-methyl-para-tyrosine, alpha-methyl-dopa, lithium, amiodarone, phenelzine (rare)
Parkinson-plus syndromes	**Progressive supranuclear palsy (PSP)** **Multiple system atrophy (MSA)** – also known as: (a) Sporadic olivopontine cerebellar atrophy (OPCA) (b) Shy–Drager syndrome (c) Striatonigral degeneration (SND)

TABLE 10.1 (*Cont'd*)	
Causes of secondary parkinsonism	**Examples**
Other degenerative diseases	Corticobasal degeneration Alzheimer's and Pick's diseases Creutzfeldt–Jakob disease
Other CNS disorders	**Multiple cerebral infarction** Hydrocephalus (normal and high pressure) Brain tumours and arteriovenous malformations Post-traumatic encephalopathy Electrical injury, subdural haematoma
Metabolic conditions	Disorders of calcium metabolism (with or without basal ganglia calcification) Chronic hepatocerebral degeneration
Hereditary disorders	Wilson's disease Huntington's disease (rigid variant)

10.2 What is a Parkinson-plus syndrome?

A neurodegenerative disorder in which the loss of the dopaminergic nigrostriatal pathway is only part of a more widespread degenerative process.

Parkinson-plus syndromes refer to conditions in which parkinsonism is seen in the context of other neurological problems owing to degeneration in a number of CNS systems. The variable extent to which these systems are affected dictates the symptoms that are experienced by the patient. Therefore patients with Parkinson-plus conditions with autonomic nervous system involvement often present with difficulties in sexual function, controlling their blood pressure and bladder; patients with cerebellar involvement often present with difficulties in controlling their balance; patients with pyramidal tract involvement have profound spasticity in the legs and arms; and patients with cortical degeneration present with marked problems with thinking that may progress to dementia.

No diagnostic test is currently available for 'idiopathic' Parkinson's disease; therefore resolving which diagnosis a patient is suffering from may be difficult, especially as many of the Parkinson-plus syndromes also do not have diagnostic tests. As a result, clinicians must very commonly rely on their experience and clinical acumen to distinguish these diagnostic problems.

10.3   Is misdiagnosis of Parkinson-plus syndromes common?

Yes, misdiagnosis of PD occurs in about 10–20% of cases.

Research has been performed to compare the clinical details and diagnoses made during a patient's lifetime with the pathological findings of the patient's brain at post-mortem. This research has shown that the misdiagnosis of Parkinson's disease in patients with Parkinson-plus syndromes is not rare. In well-established neurological centres misdiagnosis rates of over 10% have been recorded, and the rate of misdiagnosis is much higher at the time of disease onset. Similarly, studies have also shown that a significant proportion of cases of disease classified as being Parkinson-plus syndrome during life have had pathological findings of true Parkinson's disease at post-mortem.

10.4   Is misdiagnosis of Parkinson-plus syndromes clinically important?

Yes, not only because it is important to get the diagnosis correct but because it influences treatment and prognosis.

Certain parkinsonian syndromes do have specific therapeutic approaches that are highly beneficial and in these cases misdiagnosis is naturally of great consequence. For example, placement of a ventriculo-peritoneal shunt may relieve symptoms in patients with 'normal pressure hydrocephalus', and certain neoplasms may be treated with surgery, radiotherapy or chemotherapy. Cessation of the offending drugs may improve or prevent further deterioration in patients with drug-induced parkinsonism.

Accurate diagnosis is also vital for information regarding prognosis and therapeutic strategies. Although it is true that certain Parkinson-plus syndromes are responsive (often transiently) to standard Parkinson's disease therapy (e.g. progressive supranuclear palsy, multiple system atrophy) this is usually to a much lesser extent than seen in Parkinson's disease. Furthermore, those same treatments can in certain instances lead to an exacerbation of symptoms, such as the induction of more florid hallucinations in Lewy body dementia (*see* Q. *3.3*). It must be remembered that postural hypotension in a parkinsonian patient may be due either to excessive drug therapy with L-dopa or dopamine agonists but may also indicate a diagnosis such as multiple system atrophy with autonomic nervous system involvement. Finally, at a time when the possibility of curative neural transplantation techniques is being investigated, correct identification of the target population is becoming even more critical.

10.5   When should a Parkinson-plus syndrome be considered as a diagnosis?

Symmetrical onset of a poorly L-dopa responsive condition with signs that indicate significant involvement of systems other than the nigrostriatal dopaminergic pathway.

It is probably worth remembering that most of these conditions, like true Parkinson's disease, represent progressive neurological disorders. As such, the typical features of any of these syndromes may not be apparent at the initial onset of disease. When in doubt about a patient's evolving symptoms, it is often best to continue to investigate the patient and be prepared to re-evaluate the clinical diagnosis. This is best approached with an open and inclusive policy that includes the patient and the patient's family and carers. Committing early to an erroneous diagnosis tends to cause more problems than an honest disclosure of uncertainty.

Features suggesting a Parkinson-plus syndrome are included in Table 10.2.

TABLE 10.2   Symptoms and suggestions to help in the diagnosis of Parkinson-plus syndromes

Symptom	Diagnosis to consider	Practical hints
Unexplained falling early in disease course, especially on turning	Progressive supranuclear palsy	Look for full range of eye movements – loss of downgaze is suggestive of PSP (loss of upgaze is common in the normal elderly population)
Double or blurred vision	Progressive supranuclear palsy	Look for full range of eye movements (Snellen chart examination is usually normal)
Prolonged or excessive dizziness on standing	Multiple system atrophy	Check postural blood pressure
Unsteady walking 'as if drunk'	Multiple system atrophy	Check for other cerebellar signs such as finger–nose ataxia or past pointing
Bladder or sexual dysfunction	Multiple system atrophy	Assess bladder function with urodynamic studies
Cognitive problems or hallucinations especially soon after starting dopaminergic therapy	Dementia with Lewy bodies	Consider drug/infection or metabolic cause

TABLE 10.2 *(Cont'd)*

Symptom	Diagnosis to consider	Practical hints
Dyspraxia/alien hand phenomenon (*see* Q. 10.8)	Corticobasal degeneration	Follow up in specialist clinic
No response to L-dopa	Any of the above	Ensure trial of adequate dose
Other neurological abnormality, e.g. difficulty with speech or swallowing	Any of the above	Refer to speech and language therapist

10.6 What is progressive supranuclear palsy?

A neurodegenerative condition of unknown aetiology that is characterised by axial rigidity, loss of eye movements, and a frontal dementia.

Progressive supranuclear palsy (PSP) was originally described by three Canadian doctors, Steele, Richardson, and Olszewski, in the 1960s and is a progressive neurodegenerative condition. It is the disease that is most commonly confused with idiopathic Parkinson's disease as evidenced by clinicopathological reviews. The clinical features of PSP are presented in Box 10.1.

BOX 10.1 The clinical features associated with PSP

Clinical features of PSP

Disease onset is most frequently in the sixth decade with:

- *Balance disturbance*
  - Sudden unexplained falls, usually backwards are the commonest first symptom, often as the patient is turning.
- *Trouble with eyesight*
  - Usually later than the balance problems, with the earliest difficulties being most frequently in reading, owing to an inability to control downward gaze.
  - Difficulty with sustained eye contact.
  - Difficulty walking downstairs.
  - There is eventually loss in all voluntary eye movements but the ability to fixate vision during passive head movements is maintained (so-called intact doll's-eye movements – or the oculocephalic reflex).
- *Disturbance of speech and swallowing*
  - Slurring and reduced volume of speech, and eventually many patients become mute.
  - Aspiration of liquids prior to difficulty with solids.

> **BOX 10.1 (Cont'd)**
>
> ■ *Mild frontal-type dementia*
> A lack of resting tremor, symmetrical onset and axial rigidity (i.e. neck and body) help distinguish PSP from Parkinson's disease.
>
> **Investigations of PSP**
> MRI may show atrophy of the midbrain in the region of the red nuclei and superior colliculi, although these findings are generally non-specific. PET scanning reveals reduced dopaminergic levels in the striatum but again is non-specific.

No cause has been determined for PSP but a genetic predisposition is suspected and a rare familial form of the disease exists. It has been discovered that an abnormality of 'tau' protein can lead to the development of neurofibrillary tangles which can be seen under the microscope in the brain at post-mortem of patients dying with PSP.

As far as the practical consequences of the diagnosis go, some patients with PSP derive some benefit from treatment with L-dopa; however, this is usually slight and unsustained. (PSP patients tend not to suffer from fluctuations or dyskinesias following L-dopa treatment.) Dopamine agonists, amantadine and anticholinergic therapies may also be tried but the response is typically poor or non-existent, so supportive measures are probably more important.

These supportive measures should include adequate education, information and advice regarding the diagnosis. Family members should be told that problems with eye movements and emotions are a part of the illness and many of the problems can be intermittent. Measures to reduce the risks and hazards of falling include walking aids weighted to the front to prevent falling backwards, and handrails to stabilise walking may also be very useful. Further information regarding this condition can be found through the Society for PSP. Addresses and useful web sites for further information on PSP can be found in Chapter 11 (*Q. 11.10*).

10.7   What is multiple system atrophy?

A progressive neurodegenerative disorder of unknown aetiology which is characterised by a combination of parkinsonism, autonomic failure, cerebellar degeneration and relatively well preserved cognition.

Multiple system atrophy (MSA) is a general term for a spectrum of three disorders that all have some degree of parkinsonism as a feature, but also have other overlapping neurological signs (*Box 10.2*). Pathological examination of the brain shows extensive loss of neurons from the substantia nigra in all of these disorders but with an absence of Lewy

---

BOX 10.2 The three clinical variants of MSA

Clinical variants

Striatonigral degeneration (SND)
■ Predominantly akinetic–rigid parkinsonian features
■ Poor L-dopa responsiveness
■ No dementia
■ No significant autonomic or cerebellar disturbances

Shy–Drager syndrome
■ Predominant autonomic dysfunction
■ Orthostatic hypotension
■ Urinary incontinence or retention
■ Erectile impairment
■ Loss of sweating
■ Laryngeal stridor or snoring
■ Mild motor symptoms

Olivo-ponto-cerebellar atrophy (OPCA)
■ Predominant balance coordination and speech difficulties

Useful investigations for MSA patients
■ Lying–standing blood pressure and pulse
■ Formal tilt table testing
■ External sphincter electromyography

---

bodies. α-synuclein-positive inclusion bodies may, however, be seen within glial cells called oligodendrocytes. Neuronal loss in other systems correlates with the clinical picture, e.g. cerebellar ataxia relates to degeneration of the tracts between the cerebellum and brainstem, and postural hypotension is seen with degeneration occurring within the spinal cord and brainstem autonomic nuclei.

All of the variants of MSA tend to present in middle age but never before the age of 40. Standard Parkinson's disease treatment usually causes little improvement in the clinical picture, but in some cases a marked response can be seen, although this is often only transient. It is important, though, to closely monitor the response since the treatment may make things worse, e.g. dizziness due to worsening orthostatic hypotension is often exacerbated by L-dopa. Fludrocortisone or midodrine may be successful in managing difficulties in blood pressure, if simple measures such as support stockings and elevating the head end of the bed prove unhelpful. Detrusor instability can sometimes be managed successfully with peripherally acting anticholinergic agents such as oxybutynin, or intermittent/indwelling catheterisation. Ataxia has been helped modestly in some cases by the addition of amantadine.

As with all the Parkinson-plus syndromes, it is important to identify those problems which are most interfering with the patient's quality of life and attempt to find practical solutions for them.

No causes of MSA have been identified except for a familial form of OPCA. The mean survival of patients with MSA is about 8–10 years from presentation. No diagnostic test exists for MSA but dominant autonomic or cerebellar symptoms in a poorly L-dopa responsive parkinsonian patient should arouse the suspicion of MSA. In some centres an EMG of the external sphincter can be done and this is typically abnormal in MSA, although again is not specific for the condition.

10.8   What is corticobasal degeneration?

A very rare neurodegenerative condition of unknown aetiology which is characterised by parkinsonism, sensory disturbance, dyspraxia and cognitive difficulties.

This disease is famous for presenting as the 'alien hand syndrome'. Corticobasal degeneration (CBD) represents a very rare Parkinson-plus condition, the cause of which is again not known. There is progressive degeneration of both the brain's cortex and the basal ganglia, with symptoms beginning at or around age 60.

The alien hand phenomenon is another form of apraxia in which patients may have no control over a hand which appears to observers to be moving appropriately. The clinical features of CBD are summarised in Box 10.3. No drug therapies have been shown to benefit the symptoms of this condition, although clonazepam may help troublesome myoclonus. Patients usually die of medical complications of the disease 6–8 years after diagnosis.

BOX 10.3   Clinical features of CBD

Clinical features

- *Asymmetrical parkinsonism* – including rigidity, akinesia, postural instability and poor coordination.
- *Progressive apraxia* – the alien hand syndrome which may become bilateral.

Myoclonus, sensory loss, cognitive impairment and dysphagia are other recognised features. The patient is frequently unable to walk with advanced disease.

Investigations

MRI may reveal asymmetrical cerebral and pontine atrophy.

10.9 Which medications cause parkinsonism?

Many, but especially antipsychotics (major tranquillisers) and antiemetics such as metoclopramide and prochlorperazine.

It is well known that commonly used antipsychotic medications (phenothiazines and butyrophenones) inhibit all of the brain's dopaminergic neurotransmitter systems and in certain individuals can give rise to parkinsonism. The frequently used antiemetic drugs metoclopramide (Maxolon), and prochlorperazine (Stemetil), can also cause symptoms of parkinsonism in some patients. Symptoms can develop irrespective of the age of the patient and are not related to the duration of treatment.

Patients with drug-induced parkinsonism tend to have symmetrical disease that mainly affects the upper limbs. Disturbance of gait and freezing are rare.

Many other medications are known to produce symptoms such as tremor (e.g. sodium valproate, lithium) and their withdrawal usually improves these features, although this recovery may take several months. It is also worth noting that latent Parkinson's disease may be uncovered by the administration of such medications (*see also Table 10.1*).

Drug-induced movement disorders are listed in Table 10.3.

TABLE 10.3 Drug-induced movement disorders

Movement disorder	Commonly associated drugs
Tremor	Bronchodilators Lithium Valproate Caffeine Alcohol withdrawal
Parkinsonism	Neuroleptics
Acute dystonic reactions	Metoclopramide
Chorea + tardive dyskinesia	Prochlorperazine
Dyskinesias	Neuroleptics Prolonged use of dopaminergic agents
Akathisia	Neuroleptics Metoclopramide Prochlorperazine Tetrabenazine
Tics	L-dopa
Myoclonus	Dopamine agonists Anticonvulsants

10.10 Do any toxins cause parkinsonism?

Yes, a few, but such cases are rare.

Carbon monoxide (CO) poisoning has been associated with the development of an acute parkinsonian syndrome following a single exposure. This can also occur after an initial recovery and a delay of a few weeks in patients with severe CO poisoning. Heavy metals such as cobalt and manganese have been associated with similar syndromes following prolonged exposure and the association is seen typically in the context of miners working with the ore.

10.11 Can strokes cause parkinsonism?

Yes, about 3–6% of cases of parkinsonism are due to this.

Approximately 3–6% of all cases of parkinsonism have a vascular cause. In addition, features of parkinsonism are also seen in up to 38% of stroke patients 1 year after their stroke. During a patient assessment, a vascular cause for parkinsonism may be suggested by an acute onset of symptoms or a history of completed strokes. In addition, finding parkinsonism in the absence of resting tremor, or the presence of pyramidal signs, or dementia, is also suggestive of this diagnosis although these findings are certainly not invariable. 'Lower body parkinsonism' describes patients with minimal upper limb involvement and gait disturbance, and is also accepted by some as being normally due to a vascular form of parkinsonism (VP).

Patients suspected of vascular parkinsonism should undergo brain imaging to support the diagnosis, although many patients with genuine Parkinson's disease also have coincidental vascular lesions seen on their brain scans. CT detects the larger lacunes of the basal ganglia but not those in the thalamus and often not those in the brainstem. The more recent use of MRI has led to the description of 'white matter hyperintensities'. These abnormalities have been divided into either deep confluent lesions, irregular periventricular lesions (both related to arteriosclerotic disease) or periventricular lesions with smooth halos (related to demyelination and gliosis). All have been implicated in the development of vascular parkinsonism.

It seems reasonable to adopt the terms 'possible VP' for a patient with parkinsonian symptoms and a history of stroke together with striatal or extrastriatal vascular lesions on imaging, and 'probable VP' where the spatial and temporal development of lesions and symptoms are concretely linked. Post-mortem studies confirm that neuropathological examination remains the standard for making a 'definite' diagnosis of both VP and IPD.

Patients with parkinsonism secondary to strokes have a lower overall responsiveness to L-dopa, although almost all studies find that *some* VP patients will respond to L-dopa; therefore an adequate trial of L-dopa therapy should be attempted. Antiplatelet treatments may also help prevent further progression of symptoms, and it is important to address the vascular risk factors such as hypertension in these patients.

10.12 Are there any inherited causes of parkinsonian syndromes?

Yes, but normally only in young patients (i.e. those under the age of 30 years at presentation).

The important differential diagnosis of inherited disorders that mimic Parkinson's disease should be considered in any patient with a young-onset presentation. Wilson's disease is an autosomal recessive abnormality of copper metabolism which can be readily diagnosed by tests for serum copper and caeruloplasmin, and is treatable. Other inherited conditions such as Huntington's disease, the spinocerebellar ataxias, and the leukodystrophies must be diagnosed to appropriately advise family members regarding heritable risks. In addition, familial forms of PD exist which can sometimes present in a slightly atypical fashion (*see Q. 1.15*).

10.13 Can infections cause parkinsonism?

Very rarely, yes.

The classical example of this infectious parkinsonism is the 'post-encephalitic parkinsonism' (encephalitis lethargica) seen following the influenza pandemic in the early part of the 20th century. This type of disease is now incredibly rare. Japanese B encephalitis is, however, still a common problem in Asia, and parkinsonism is not infrequently seen during the acute illness. There is usually spontaneous improvement in akinesia and rigidity following resolution of the illness; however, dystonia can frequently remain a problem.

The new variant of Creutzfeldt–Jakob disease (vCJD), due to the transmissible prion protein that causes bovine spongiform encephalopathy (BSE), has been shown to demonstrate a wide variety of neurological features, including parkinsonism. Patients with vCJD tend to have cerebellar signs, myoclonus or dementia, but it remains a very rare diagnosis at the current time.

Up to 40% of AIDS patients develop subtle signs of parkinsonism. Symptoms may occur as part of an HIV encephalopathy, secondary to opportunistic infections or CNS lymphoma. Treatment should be directed at the underlying cause. HIV parkinsonism tends to be unresponsive to L-dopa.

10.14 Can cerebral mass lesions cause parkinsonism?

Yes, but this is an unusual presentation for cerebral mass lesions.

A tumour (e.g. lymphoma) located either in the parasagittal area or in the upper brainstem, or any space-occupying lesion leading to obstructive hydrocephalus may cause parkinsonism. The possibility of a cerebral mass lesion should be suspected if there are any atypical features, especially features suggestive of raised intracranial pressure such as postural headache, vomiting or papilloedema. Likewise, a patient with normal pressure hydrocephalus (characterised by gait disturbance, dementia and incontinence) must be identified for consideration of shunt insertion. Diagnosis is straightforward, with either CT or MRI scanning identifying the majority of cerebral mass lesions. The prognosis for cerebral mass lesions depends on the precise location and on the underlying histology.

10.15 What is essential tremor?

A relatively common condition, often familial, that is characterised by a postural tremor of limbs, head and voice, but with no other parkinsonian features.

Essential tremor is another common neurological disorder in which the patient may have a tremor affecting the hands, head, legs, trunk or voice. The underlying pathophysiology is unknown, and no structural brain lesion has been identified. A family history is quite common in this disorder and two genetic loci responsible for some cases of ET have been identified. The tremor tends to be symmetrical and patients sometimes have an improvement in their symptoms following alcohol. This type of tremor is often referred to as 'benign' but in some cases can be quite disabling. In a minority of cases, the patient may develop other extrapyramidal symptoms such as bradykinesia years later. Whether there is a genuine link between ET and Parkinson's disease requires further study. Treatments with β-blockers such as propranolol 80 mg b.d., or primidone 50 mg o.d., are often beneficial for ET, and in severe cases, thalamotomy, or thalamic deep brain stimulation are used (*see Ch. 8*).

10.16 What is dystonic tremor?

An unusual condition in which a part of the body is held in an abnormal posture (dystonia) and rhythmically shakes (tremor).

Tremor and dystonia occasionally coexist in patients who do not show any other symptoms of Parkinson's disease and who have never been exposed to dopaminergic medications. The tremor and dystonia may both affect the same part of the body, e.g. one particular limb or the neck, or they may occur in distinct places. The relationship of this form of tremor to essential tremor or PD is not known.

PQ PATIENT QUESTIONS

The consultant says I have MSA – what is that?

MSA stands for multiple system atrophy and is a rare condition that affects the brain. Most people with MSA have symptoms of Parkinson's disease, but also have other symptoms because other brain 'systems' are also affected. This is why you have problems with your bladder/blood pressure/breathing/ balance control.

The consultant says I have PSP – what is that?

PSP stands for progressive supranuclear palsy and is a condition separate from Parkinson's disease but which causes symptoms similar to it, as well as causing falls and difficulties with moving your eyes. This is why you have difficulty when you are walking downstairs. The name 'supranuclear palsy' refers to the damaged system in the brain above or 'supra' to the 'nuclei' which normally control eye movements.

Could my parkinsonism be due to strokes?

It is *possible* for strokes or 'mini-strokes' to cause symptoms similar to Parkinson's disease, but this is unusual and when it does happen, patients usually have sudden changes in their symptoms rather than a gradual progression. Strokes usually cause other symptoms in addition to the ones of Parkinson's disease, which you do not have, and therefore it seems unlikely that strokes are causing your symptoms.

Sources of further information and support

11.1 How can the Internet help in Parkinson's disease?

By providing useful information from recognised well-informed web sites.

The Internet is a valuable and frequent source of information for patients and doctors alike. It is important that patients do not become misinformed about their disease by reading information from unreliable Internet sources, and we have therefore included recommended Internet web site addresses within this chapter.

The Internet is also a valuable method of communication and correspondence especially for people who may have difficulty with movements, walking, writing and even speech.

11.2 What web sites are useful for further education in Parkinson's disease?

A list of addresses of web sites recommended for obtaining online information about Parkinson's disease is given below. Many of them feature links to further sources of information. Some of these sites are designed primarily for patients, some for doctors and researchers and some for both.

The Parkinson's Disease Society
www.parkinsons.org.uk

The PDS web site gives basic information about the disease that is written in simple terms to help patients to understand. The web site provides news about the disease and details of how to join or contact the PDS.

Awakenings
www.parkinsonsdisease.com

This international site provides excellent access to information for primary care physicians, patients and specialists. Addresses and contact details of support groups are listed by country.

The site also lists some useful 'Frequently Asked Questions' from patients, and articles written by patients with young-onset PD.

We Move
www.wemove.org

Predominantly an educational site for PD as well as other movement disorders, this is a very user-friendly web site that also includes information for patients with the more obscure syndromes.

YAPP&Rs
www.yappars-parkinsons.org.uk

National Library of Medicine
www.nlm.nih.gov/medlineplus/parkinsonsdisease

This is the US National Library's web site, which includes comprehensive information on PD, news, overviews, and advice about the disease for patients. The site also includes links to explain medical terms used in PD.

The European Parkinson's Disease Association
www.shef.ac.uk/misc/groups/epda

The EPDA web site is designed to give information for those active in PD projects. The site gives notices of international conferences and meetings on PD, gives access to the EPDA newsletter on line, provides updates on projects with which the organisation is involved and has links to PD associations and societies throughout Europe.

World PD Association
www.wpda.org

The World PD Association web site has an emphasis on academic publications of interest to those with special interests in PD. The site also has PD news, health tips, and updates on PD research.

Special Parkinson's Research Interest Group
http://spring.parkinsons.org.uk

SPRING is the official Special Interest Group for Medical Research, constituted within the Parkinson's Disease Society of the UK. The aim of this site is to make research reports more intelligible to non-medically trained readers.

11.3 What organisations offer support for Parkinson's disease patients?

The Parkinson's Disease Society primarily.

Patients, their families, friends, and carers may all require support during the progression of Parkinson's disease. The diagnosis may have a significant impact on the psychosocial framework surrounding a patient, and it is important to ensure that communication is maintained and responsibilities negotiated between all the members of a patient's social framework.

There is little doubt that increasing people's understanding and awareness of their medical condition can reduce anxiety and mood disturbance as well as translate into better control. Psychosocial support, especially around the time of initial diagnosis is likely to be of great importance and, if possible, involvement of a Parkinson's disease specialist nurse is a useful first step in this counselling process. Patients may derive great support from interaction with other people with similar symptoms, and the Parkinson's Disease Society (*see* Q. *11.5*) offers the main source for support for PD patients. Further general support can be gained through a variety of agencies, the contact details for some of which are given below:

PARKINSON'S DISEASE SOCIETY OF THE UNITED KINGDOM
215 Vauxhall Bridge Road
London
SW1V 1EJ
Helpline: 0808 800 0303
www.parkinsons.org.uk

The Parkinson's Disease Society is the UK support group for patients with Parkinson's disease. It encourages both patients and carers to attend meetings at which there are opportunities to discuss the problems and limitations caused by PD and solutions to these problems.

AGE CONCERN
Astral House
1268 London Road
London
SW16 4ER
Tel: 020 8765 7200
www.ageconcern.org.uk

Age Concern provides advice for patients and carers and help in locating local support groups and services, including day centres, lunch clubs, home visits and transport services.

BRITISH ASSOCIATION OF COUNSELLING
1 Regent Place
Rugby
Warwickshire
CV21 2PJ
Tel: 01788 550 899
www.bac.co.uk

This organisation provides help in finding counsellors, psychotherapists, and related charities and organisations within a patient's area. Additional information may also be given, such as the services offered, qualifications, clientele, and fees.

THE CONTINENCE FOUNDATION
307 Hatton Square
16 Baldwin Gardens
London
EC1N 7RL
Helpline: 020 7831 9831
www.continence-foundation.org.uk

The foundation provides information about bladder and bowel problems, with diagrams; and information on products, with illustrations and advice on choices for the general public.

COUNSEL AND CARE
Twyman House
16 Bonny Street
London
NW1 9PG
Tel: 0845 300 7585
www.counselandcare.org.uk

Access to advice and information for older people (60 and over) living in the UK is provided through fact sheets and email, including details of welfare benefits and sources of help for paying for community care.

RELATE
(Counselling for Individuals and Couples)
Tel: 01788 573 241
www.relate.org.uk

Relate is the relationship counselling organisation in the UK.

SPOD
(Association to aid the Sexual and Personal Relationships of People with a Disability)
286 Camden Road
London
N7 0BJ
Tel: 020 7607 8851
www.spod-uk.org

SPOD publish and sell several information leaflets on a range of sexuality and relationship issues for disabled people. The online versions are free to view in the members' area.

If the stress of the illness exceeds the coping strategies of the patient or caregivers, a referral may be made for psychological counselling. It is also important to consider the possibility of depression in patients struggling to come to terms with their diagnosis (*see Qs 3.11 and 6.10*).

11.4 Where can carers of Parkinson's disease patients get support?

From a number of sources (*see Q. 11.3*).

The Parkinson's Disease Society welcomes carers for patients with Parkinson's disease to attend meetings and discuss problems that they face as a result of the disease. There are also associations specifically for carers of people with disabilities. The Crossroads scheme 'Caring for Carers' has over 200 schemes across England and Wales providing carers with high-quality support. Trained care workers go into the home and take over the caring tasks, enabling the carer to go shopping, have some free time or even catch up with sleep. The Crossroads scheme can be found at:

Crossroads
10 Regent Place
Rugby
Warwickshire
CV21 2PN
01788 573653
www.crossroads.org.uk

11.5 What is the Parkinson's Disease Society?

A society founded in the 1960s, that supports patients and their carers as well as funding research and welfare support.

The Parkinson's Disease Society (PDS) was founded in 1969 and is now the main source of help to people with Parkinson's disease in the UK. In addition to its own branches, it can put patients in touch with many other sources of practical help and advice. The founder members of PDS were people with Parkinson's disease, relatives and friends who provided information written in layman's language for other sufferers of the disease. Membership of the society costs only £4.00 per year.
  Services offered by the society include:
■ A newsletter, 'The Parkinson', published four times a year
■ Many helpful booklets, tapes and videos
■ A publication list
■ Regular meetings as a source of sharing information and support.
  The society can be contacted in writing or online at:

Parkinson's Disease Society of the United Kingdom
215 Vauxhall Bridge Road
London
SW1V 1EJ
Tel: 020 7931 8080
Helpline: 0808 800 0303 (Monday–Friday, 09.30–17.30)
Fax: 020 7233 9908
www.parkinsons.org.uk

Parkinson's Disease Society Office in Scotland
10 Claremont Terrace
Glasgow
G3 7XR
Tel/fax: 0141 332 3343

The PDS also has a special section called 'Young Alert Parkinson's, Partners and Relatives' (YAPP&Rs) for younger people with Parkinson's disease (*see Q. 11.6*).

11.6　What is YAPP&Rs?

A special section of the PDS designed to help younger patients with PD.

YAPP&Rs is the 'Young Alert Parkinson's, Partners and Relatives' self-help support group of the Parkinson's Disease Society of the UK. It is a special interest group for people with Parkinson's disease and their families who are of 'working age' and below.

This subsidiary body of the PDS was established because of the different problems experienced by people with PD occurring at a younger age, including:

- family relationships, particularly in connection with children
- employment and the possibility of early retirement
- concerns about mortgages and other financial matters.

The YAPP&Rs meetings allow younger people with PD, who want to meet others with young-onset PD, and their carers, an opportunity to share experiences and offer each other support. There are at present 18 groups around the UK.

YAPP&Rs produce their own quarterly magazine, called the *YAPmag*.

Further details can be obtained from:

YAPP&Rs
YAPMAIL
PO Box 33209
London
SW1V 1WH
Tel: 0808 800 0303 (PDS national helpline number)
www.yappars-parkinsons.org.uk

11.7   Where can patients get more advice on disabilities?

Sources of information, advice and aids for people with disabilities are given below (*see also* Q. *11.3*).

THE DISABLED LIVING FOUNDATION

380–384 Harrow Road
London
W9 2HU
Tel: 0845 130 9177
www.dlf.org.uk

The web site provides superb access to descriptions of the range of equipment available, with certain items available for order online, or contact details for suppliers.

THE DISABLED LIVING CENTRES COUNCIL

1st Floor
Winchester House
11 Cranmer Road
Kennington
London
SW9 6EJ
Tel: 020 7820 0567
www.dlcc.co.uk

The council provides information and advice about products that can increase disabled or older people's choices about how they live. They provide opportunities to see and try out products and explore other solutions.

DISABLED LIVING

4 St Chad's Street
Cheetham
Manchester
M8 8QA
Tel: 0161 214 5959
www.disabledliving.co.uk

The web site provides information on products, holidays, clothes, etc. which are disabled friendly, and where to get them. There is also advice and information on products which help with daily living including advice on suppliers and prices.

KEEP ABLE
Sterling Park
Pedmore Road
Brierley Hill
W. Midlands
DY5 1TB
Tel: 08705 202122
www.keepable.co.uk

Keep Able is a commercial company involved in the sale of many useful products for the disabled. They will perform home assessments, and have a mail order catalogue. There are branches in London, Staines, Kettering, Bristol, Brierley Hill and Worcester.

11.8 What are the best reference papers for specific aspects of Parkinson's disease?

It is almost impossible to keep up with the enormous wealth of literature published from one year to the next on the many aspects of Parkinson's disease. Good sources for further reading for some of the different aspects of PD are listed below:

EPIDEMIOLOGY

Tanner CM, Ben Shlomo Y 1999 Epidemiology of Parkinson's disease. *Advances in Neurology* 80: 153–159

GENETICS

Gasser T 1999 Is Parkinson's disease an inherited condition? *Advances in Neurology* 80: 143–152

PATHOLOGY

Hughes AJ, Daniel SE, Blankson S, Lees AJ 1993 A clinicopathologic study of 100 cases of Parkinson's disease. *Archives of Neurology* 50: 140–148

CLINICAL FEATURES

Hoehn MM, Yahr MD 1967 Parkinsonism: onset, progression and mortality. *Neurology* 17: 427–442

DIAGNOSIS

Brooks DJ 2000 Morphological and functional imaging studies on the diagnosis and progression of Parkinson's disease. *Journal of Neurology* 247 (Suppl 2): II11–II18
Koller WC, Montgomery EB 1997 Issues in the early diagnosis of Parkinson's disease. *Neurology* 49: S10–S25

COGNITION

Owen AM, James M, Leigh PN, Summers BA, Marsden CD, Quinn NP et al 1992 Fronto-striatal cognitive deficits at different stages of Parkinson's disease. *Brain* 115: 1727–1751

MANAGEMENT

Deep-Brain Stimulation for Parkinson's Disease Study Group 2001 Deep-brain stimulation of the subthalamic nucleus or the pars interna of the globus pallidus in Parkinson's disease. *New England Journal of Medicine* 345(13): 956–963

Miyasaki JM, Martin W, Sucherowsky O, Weiner WJ, Lang AE 2002 Practice parameter: initiation of treatment for Parkinson's disease: an evidence based review. *Neurology* 58: 11–17

Olanow CW, Watts RL, Koller WC 2001 An algorithm (decision tree) for the management of Parkinson's disease (2001): treatment guidelines. *Neurology* 56: S1–S88

α-SYNUCLEIN

Goedert M 2001 Alpha-synuclein and neurodegenerative diseases. *Nature Reviews Neuroscience* 2: 492–501

11.9 **What sources of further general reading are recommended for Parkinson's disease?**

An excellent overview of many aspects of Parkinson's disease written by Anthony Lang and Andres Lozano was published in two parts in the *New England Journal of Medicine* in 1998 (Vol 339: 1044–1053 and 1130–1143).

Some other recommended books on PD include the following:

■ *The Comprehensive Management of Parkinson's Disease* (AM Cohen and W J Weiner, 1994, Demos Publications, New York)
■ *Parkinson's at Your Fingertips* (M Oxtoby and A Williams, 1997, Class Publishing, London)
■ *Awakenings* (O Sacks, 1982, Picador, London).

11.10 **Where can I find out more for people with Parkinson-plus syndromes?**

Contact details for societies that provide information and support for Parkinson-plus sufferers are given below:

PROGRESSIVE SUPRANUCLEAR PALSY

The PSP Association
The Outbuildings
The Old Rectory

Wappenham
Nr Towcester
Northamptonshire
NN12 8SQ
Tel: 01327 860299
www.cafamily.org.uk

The PSP Association is a registered national charity established by a patient with PSP, and acts as a UK support group. The association publishes a newsletter and holds meetings for both patients and researchers of the disease. More information about the association and links to the European PSP association can be found through their web site.

The Society for Progressive Supranuclear Palsy
Woodholme Medical Building
Suite 515
1838 Greene Tree Road
Baltimore, MD
USA 21208
www.psp.org

The Society for PSP has a useful web site for fact sheets about PSP, with news and research about the disease and links to other sites.

MULTIPLE SYSTEM ATROPHY
The Autonomic Disorders Association
Sarah Matheson Trust
St Mary's Hospital
Praed St
London
W2 1NY
Tel: 020 7886 1520

The Autonomic Disorders Association provides patients with information and an opportunity to meet other MSA sufferers.

National Dysautonomia Research Foundation
421 West Fourth Street
Suite 9
Red Wing, MN
USA 55066-2555
www.ndrf.org

More information on MSA can be found on the movement disorders web site:
www.wemove.org/msa

11.11 Does any research offer hope for Parkinson's disease patients of the future?

Most definitely yes.

The latest research in Parkinson's disease is offering considerable hope for greater understanding of the causes of PD. Understanding the role of the cellular proteosome system in the metabolism of abnormal proteins may provide the link between a host of possible environmental and genetic risks for PD. Once this system is understood, disease prevention, neuro-protection and neuro-rescue may be feasible approaches in conquering PD and other neurodegenerative diseases.

In the meantime, surgical treatments, especially deep brain stimulators may soon offer many more patients good long-term symptom control. Furthermore, it is clear that cell transplants from several sources can survive within the PD brain and produce new functional dopamine-producing neurons, and these transplants may yet offer a curative PD treatment.

11.12 Are any other drugs on the horizon of possible benefit for Parkinson's disease?

A few, but the long-acting dopamine agonists are probably the best option at the moment.

It is believed that the development of dyskinesias may be hastened by pulsatile stimulation of dopamine receptors, and as a result there is much interest in therapies that reduce the pulsatility of dopaminergic stimulation. The main focus has been on long-acting dopamine agonists (pergolide, ropinirole, pramipexole, and cabergoline) (*see Qs 5.6 and 5.7*).

In addition, however, two trials of opioid antagonists have shown improvements in dyskinesias experienced by PD patients without deterioration in their other symptoms, although these findings need further confirmation. Other promising results have also been reported in studies of adenosine A2A ligands, α_2-adrenoceptor antagonists, and novel 5-HT agonists, but large-scale clinical trials have yet to be conducted.

A small number of patients have been treated with an infusion of a substance called glial derived neurotrophic factor (GDNF) directly into the affected areas of the brain. Some of those treated have reported a beneficial response to this therapy, which has generated a lot of publicity. While it is certainly encouraging, it is important that these findings are repeated in larger, placebo-controlled trials before conclusions can be reached on the usefulness of the treatment.

PQ PATIENT QUESTIONS

Should I join the PDS as I'm worried about seeing how bad some patients with Parkinson's disease can be?

It is natural for you to be a little worried about meeting other people with Parkinson's disease for the first time, especially while your own symptoms are comparatively mild. The Parkinson's Disease Society, however, is a source of support for all people coping with Parkinson's disease and you may even find it difficult to spot which members of any group have the illness and which are the carers. People who have had the disease for many years are often a valuable source of information and tips about how to cope with aspects of the disease that even the specialists are not aware of.

Before launching yourself into the PD society, it would be sensible to read some of their literature, and ask for information about the PDS groups in your area. If one group is not suited to you, then you may find greater support through another, especially if you have young-onset disease, as a special support group exists for such patients (YAPP&Rs – *see Q. 11.6*). Remember that the illness can affect different people in different ways, and no-one can predict how slow or fast the disease will progress in any individual.

REFERENCES

Chapter 1

1. Hoehn MM, Yahr MD 1967 Parkinsonism: onset, progression and mortality. *Neurology* 17: 427–442
2. Parkinson J 1817 *An essay on the shaking palsy.* Whittingham and Rowland, London

Chapter 2

1. Johns MW 1991 A new method for measuring daytime sleepiness: the Epworth sleepiness scale. *Sleep* 14: 540–545

Chapter 4

1. Benamer HTS, Patterson J, Grosset DG et al 2000 Accurate differentiation of parkinsonism and essential tremor using visual assessment of [^{123}I]-FP-CIT-SPECT imaging: the [^{123}I]-FP-CIT Study Group. *Movement Disorders* 15(3): 503–510

Chapter 10

1. Deuschl G, Bain P, Brin M and an Ad Hoc Scientific Committee 1998 Consensus statement of the Movement Disorder Society on tremor. *Movement Disorders* 13 (Suppl 3): 2–23

Appendix 1

1. Yesavage JA, Brink TL, Rose TL, Lum O, Huang V, Adey MB, Leirer VO 1983 Development and validation of a geriatric depression screening scale: A preliminary report. *Journal of Psychiatric Research* 17: 37–49
2. Sheikh JI, Yesavage JA 1986 Geriatric Depression Scale (GDS): Recent evidence and development of a shorter version. *Clinical Gerontology: A Guide to Assessment and Intervention* 165–173. The Haworth Press, New York

This appendix includes four rating scales that are particularly useful in assessing various aspects of Parkinson's disease. All these scales have been subjected to reliability and validity testing.

The Mini Mental State Examination (reproduced in part) is a quick way of identifying evidence of cognitive impairment.

The Unified Parkinson's Disease Rating Scale (UPDRS) allows quantification of the motor and non-motor aspects of PD and can be used to monitor progression of the disease.

The Parkinson's Disease Questionnaire (PDQ-39) addresses quality of life issues for individual PD patients, which should be a major priority for the primary care physician.

The Geriatric Depression Scale is a useful way of detecting and monitoring clinical or subclinical depression in older PD patients.

The Mini Mental State Examination

This rating scale is commonly used in medical practice and attempts to assess a wide range of cognitive processes. The scale includes the questions listed in Box A.1 and takes between 5–10 minutes to administer. The MMSE, however, takes no account of mood, thought disturbance or perception but attempts to cover areas of cognition such as orientation, memory and attention.

The scoring system gives a maximum of 30 points, and scores of 24 and above would be considered satisfactory; between 17 and 24 would suggest likely cognitive impairment and below 17 definite dementia. It should be highlighted, however, that many patients who suffer with discrete cognitive difficulties compared to healthy age-matched individuals, score well in the normal range of the MMSE, making it a less useful tool for screening milder cognitive impairment. The test is also insensitive to frontal lobe damage as is commonly seen in parkinsonian conditions.

BOX A.1 Sample items from the Mini Mental State Examination

Orientation to time
'What is the date?'

Registration
'Listen carefully, I am going to say three words. You say them back after I stop. Ready? Here they are ...
HOUSE (pause), CAR (pause), LAKE (pause). Now repeat those words back to me.'
(Repeat up to 5 times, but score only the first trial.)

Naming
'What is this?' (Point to a pen or pencil.)

Reading
'Please read this and do what it says. (Show examinee the words on the stimulus form.)
CLOSE YOUR EYES

Reproduced by special permission of the publisher, Psychological Assessment Resources, Inc., 16204 North Florida Avenue, Lutz, Florida 33549, from the Mini Mental State Examination, by Marshal Folstein and Susan Folstein. Copyright 1975, 1998, 2001 by Mini Mental LLC, Inc. Published 2001 by Psychological Assessment Resources, Inc. Further reproduction is prohibited without permission from PAR, Inc. by calling (800) 331-8378 or (813) 968-3003.

The Unified Parkinson's Disease Rating Scale (UPDRS)

Reproduced with permission of Professor Stanley Fahn.

I.   MENTATION, BEHAVIOUR AND MOOD

1. **Intellectual impairment**
   0 = None.
   1 = Mild. Consistent forgetfulness with partial recollection of events and no other difficulties.
   2 = Moderate memory loss, with disorientation and moderate difficulty handling complex problems. Mild but definite impairment of function at home with need of occasional prompting.
   3 = Severe memory loss with disorientation for time and often to place. Severe impairment in handling problems.
   4 = Severe memory loss with orientation preserved to person only. Unable to make judgements or solve problems. Requires much help with personal care. Cannot be left alone at all.

2. **Thought disorder** (due to dementia or drug intoxication)
   0 = None.
   1 = Vivid dreaming.
   2 = 'Benign' hallucinations with insight retained.
   3 = Occasional to frequent hallucinations or delusions; without insight; could interfere with daily activities.
   4 = Persistent hallucinations, delusions, or florid psychosis. Not able to care for self.

3. **Depression**
   0 = None.
   1 = Periods of sadness or guilt greater than normal, never sustained for days or weeks.
   2 = Sustained depression (1 week or more).
   3 = Sustained depression with vegetative symptoms (insomnia, anorexia, weight loss, loss of interest).
   4 = Sustained depression with vegetative symptoms and suicidal thoughts or intent.

4. **Motivation/initiative**
   0 = Normal.
   1 = Less assertive than usual; more passive.
   2 = Loss of initiative or disinterest in elective (non-routine) activities.
   3 = Loss of initiative or disinterest in day to day (routine) activities.
   4 = Withdrawn, complete loss of motivation.

II.   ACTIVITIES OF DAILY LIVING (for both 'on' and 'off')

5.   **Speech**
       0 = Normal.
       1 = Mildly affected. No difficulty being understood.
       2 = Moderately affected. Sometimes asked to repeat statements.
       3 = Severely affected. Frequently asked to repeat statements.
       4 = Unintelligible most of the time.

6.   **Salivation**
       0 = Normal.
       1 = Slight but definite excess of saliva in mouth; may have night-time drooling.
       2 = Moderately excessive saliva; may have minimal drooling.
       3 = Marked excess of saliva with some drooling.
       4 = Marked drooling, requires constant tissue or handkerchief.

7.   **Swallowing**
       0 = Normal.
       1 = Rare choking.
       2 = Occasional choking.
       3 = Requires soft food.
       4 = Requires NG tube or gastrostomy feeding.

8.   **Handwriting**
       0 = Normal.
       1 = Slightly slow or small.
       2 = Moderately slow or small; all words are legible.
       3 = Severely affected; not all words are legible.
       4 = The majority of words are not legible.

9.   **Cutting food and handling utensils**
       0 = Normal.
       1 = Somewhat slow and clumsy, but no help needed.
       2 = Can cut most foods, although clumsy and slow; some help needed.
       3 = Food must be cut by someone, but can still feed slowly.
       4 = Needs to be fed.

10.   **Dressing**
       0 = Normal.
       1 = Somewhat slow, but no help needed.
       2 = Occasional assistance with buttoning, getting arms in sleeves.
       3 = Considerable help required, but can do some things alone.
       4 = Helpless.

11.   **Hygiene**
       0 = Normal.
       1 = Somewhat slow, but no help needed.
       2 = Needs help to shower or bathe; or very slow in hygienic care.

3 = Requires assistance for washing, brushing teeth, combing hair, going to bathroom.

4 = Foley catheter or other mechanical aids.

12. Turning in bed and adjusting bedclothes

0 = Normal.

1 = Somewhat slow and clumsy, but no help needed.

2 = Can turn alone or adjust sheets, but with great difficulty.

3 = Can initiate, but not turn or adjust sheets alone.

4 = Helpless.

13. Falling (unrelated to freezing)

0 = None.

1 = Rare falling.

2 = Occasionally falls, less than once per day.

3 = Falls an average of once daily.

4 = Falls more than once daily.

14. Freezing when walking

0 = None.

1 = Rare freezing when walking; may have start hesitation.

2 = Occasional freezing when walking.

3 = Frequent freezing. Occasionally falls from freezing.

4 = Frequent falls from freezing.

15. Walking

0 = Normal.

1 = Mild difficulty. May not swing arms or may tend to drag leg.

2 = Moderate difficulty, but requires little or no assistance.

3 = Severe disturbance of walking, requiring assistance.

4 = Cannot walk at all, even with assistance.

16. Tremor (symptomatic complaint of tremor in any part of body)

0 = Absent.

1 = Slight and infrequently present.

2 = Moderate; bothersome to patient.

3 = Severe; interferes with many activities.

4 = Marked; interferes with most activities.

17. Sensory complaints related to parkinsonism

0 = None.

1 = Occasionally has numbness, tingling, or mild aching.

2 = Frequently has numbness, tingling, or aching; not distressing.

3 = Frequent painful sensations.

4 = Excruciating pain.

III. MOTOR EXAMINATION

18. Speech
0 = Normal.
1 = Slight loss of expression, diction and/or volume.
2 = Monotone, slurred but understandable; moderately impaired.
3 = Marked impairment, difficult to understand.
4 = Unintelligible.

19. Facial expression
0 = Normal.
1 = Minimal hypomimia, could be normal 'poker face'.
2 = Slight but definitely abnormal diminution of facial expression.
3 = Moderate hypomimia; lips parted some of the time.
4 = Masked or fixed facies with severe or complete loss of facial expression; lips parted $\frac{1}{4}$ inch or more.

20. Tremor at rest (head, upper and lower extremities)
0 = Absent.
1 = Slight and infrequently present.
2 = Mild in amplitude and persistent. Or moderate in amplitude, but only intermittently present.
3 = Moderate in amplitude and present most of the time.
4 = Marked in amplitude and present most of the time.

21. Action or postural tremor of hands
0 = Absent.
1 = Slight; present with action.
2 = Moderate in amplitude, present with action.
3 = Moderate in amplitude with posture holding as well as action.
4 = Marked in amplitude; interferes with feeding.

22. Rigidity (judged on passive movement of major joints with patient relaxed in sitting position; cogwheeling to be ignored)
0 = Absent.
1 = Slight or detectable only when activated by mirror or other movements.
2 = Mild to moderate.
3 = Marked, but full range of motion easily achieved.
4 = Severe, range of motion achieved with difficulty.

23. Finger taps (patient taps thumb with index finger in rapid succession)
0 = Normal.
1 = Mild slowing and/or reduction in amplitude.
2 = Moderately impaired. Definite and early fatiguing. May have occasional arrests in movement.
3 = Severely impaired. Frequent hesitation in initiating movements or arrests in ongoing movement.
4 = Can barely perform the task.

24. **Hand movements** (patient opens and closes hands in rapid succession)
     0 = Normal.
     1 = Mild slowing and/or reduction in amplitude.
     2 = Moderately impaired. Definite and early fatiguing. May have occasional arrests in movement.
     3 = Severely impaired. Frequent hesitation in initiating movements or arrests in ongoing movement.
     4 = Can barely perform the task.

25. **Rapid alternating movements of hands** (pronation–supination movements of hands, vertically and horizontally, with as large an amplitude as possible, both hands simultaneously)
     0 = Normal.
     1 = Mild slowing and/or reduction in amplitude.
     2 = Moderately impaired. Definite and early fatiguing. May have occasional arrests in movement.
     3 = Severely impaired. Frequent hesitation in initiating movements or arrests in ongoing movement.
     4 = Can barely perform the task.

26. **Leg agility** (patient taps heel on the ground in rapid succession picking up entire leg; amplitude should be at least 3 inches)
     0 = Normal.
     1 = Mild slowing and/or reduction in amplitude.
     2 = Moderately impaired. Definite and early fatiguing. May have occasional arrests in movement.
     3 = Severely impaired. Frequent hesitation in initiating movements or arrests in ongoing movement.
     4 = Can barely perform the task.

27. **Arising from chair** (patient attempts to rise from a straight-backed chair, with arms folded across chest)
     0 = Normal.
     1 = Slow; or may need more than one attempt.
     2 = Pushes self up from arms of seat.
     3 = Tends to fall back and may have to try more than one time, but can get up without help.
     4 = Unable to arise without help.

28. **Posture**
     0 = Normal erect.
     1 = Not quite erect, slightly stooped posture; could be normal for older person.
     2 = Moderately stooped posture, definitely abnormal; can be slightly leaning to one side.
     3 = Severely stooped posture with kyphosis; can be moderately leaning to one side.
     4 = Marked flexion with extreme abnormality of posture.

29. **Gait**
    0 = Normal.
    1 = Walks slowly, may shuffle with short steps, but no festination (hastening steps) or propulsion.
    2 = Walks with difficulty, but requires little or no assistance; may have some festination, short steps, or propulsion.
    3 = Severe disturbance of gait, requiring assistance.
    4 = Cannot walk at all, even with assistance.

30. **Postural stability** (response to sudden, strong posterior displacement produced by pull on shoulders while patient erect with eyes open and feet slightly apart; patient is prepared)
    0 = Normal.
    1 = Retropulsion, but recovers unaided.
    2 = Absence of postural response; would fall if not caught by examiner.
    3 = Very unstable, tends to lose balance spontaneously.
    4 = Unable to stand without assistance.

31. **Body bradykinesia and hypokinesia** (combining slowness, hesitancy, decreased armswing, small amplitude, and poverty of movement in general)
    0 = None.
    1 = Minimal slowness, giving movement a deliberate character; could be normal for some persons. Possibly reduced amplitude.
    2 = Mild degree of slowness and poverty of movement which is definitely abnormal. Alternatively, some reduced amplitude.
    3 = Moderate slowness, poverty or small amplitude of movement.
    4 = Marked slowness, poverty or small amplitude of movement.

IV. **COMPLICATIONS OF THERAPY (in the past week)**

A. *Dyskinesias*

32. **Duration: What proportion of the waking day are dyskinesias present?** (historical information)
    0 = None
    1 = 1–25% of day.
    2 = 26–50% of day.
    3 = 51–75% of day.
    4 = 76–100% of day.

33. **Disability: How disabling are the dyskinesias?** (historical information; may be modified by office examination)
    0 = Not disabling.
    1 = Mildly disabling.
    2 = Moderately disabling.
    3 = Severely disabling.
    4 = Completely disabled.

34. **Painful dyskinesias: How painful are the dyskinesias?**
    0 = No painful dyskinesias.
    1 = Slight.
    2 = Moderate.
    3 = Severe.
    4 = Marked.
35. **Presence of early morning dystonia** (historical information)
    0 = No
    1 = Yes

B. *Clinical fluctuations*

36. **Are 'off' periods predictable?**
    0 = No
    1 = Yes
37. **Are 'off' periods unpredictable?**
    0 = No
    1 = Yes
38. **Do 'off' periods come on suddenly, within a few seconds?**
    0 = No
    1 = Yes
39. **What proportion of the waking day is the patient 'off' on average?**
    0 = None.
    1 = 1–25% of day.
    2 = 26–50% of day.
    3 = 51–75% of day.
    4 = 76–100% of day.

C. *Other complications*

40. **Does the patient have anorexia, nausea, or vomiting?**
    0 = No
    1 = Yes
41. **Any sleep disturbances, such as insomnia or hypersomnolence?**
    0 = No
    1 = Yes
42. **Does the patient have symptomatic orthostasis?**
    (Record the patient's blood pressure, height and weight on the scoring form.)

The Parkinson's Disease Questionnaire (PDQ-39)

DUE TO HAVING PARKINSON'S DISEASE, how often have you experienced the following, during the last month?

Due to having Parkinson's disease, how often during the last month have you …

*Please tick **one box** for each question*

	Never	Occasionally	Sometimes	Often	Always or cannot do at all
1. Had difficulty doing the leisure activities which you would like to do?	☐	☐	☐	☐	☐
2. Had difficulty looking after your home, e.g. DIY, housework, cooking?	☐	☐	☐	☐	☐
3. Had difficulty carrying bags of shopping?	☐	☐	☐	☐	☐
4. Had problems walking half a mile?	☐	☐	☐	☐	☐
5. Had problems walking 100 yards?	☐	☐	☐	☐	☐
6. Had problems getting around the house as easily as you would like?	☐	☐	☐	☐	☐
7. Had difficulty getting around in public?	☐	☐	☐	☐	☐
8. Needed someone else to accompany you when you went out?	☐	☐	☐	☐	☐

*Please check that you have ticked **one box for each question** before going on to the next page*

Due to having Parkinson's disease, how often during the last month have you …

*Please tick **one box** for each question*

	Never	Occasionally	Sometimes	Often	Always or cannot do at all
9. Felt frightened or worried about falling over in public?	☐	☐	☐	☐	☐
10. Been confined to the house more than you would like?	☐	☐	☐	☐	☐
11. Had difficulty washing yourself?	☐	☐	☐	☐	☐
12. Had difficulty dressing yourself?	☐	☐	☐	☐	☐
13. Had problems doing up buttons or shoe laces?	☐	☐	☐	☐	☐
14. Had problems writing clearly?	☐	☐	☐	☐	☐
15. Had difficulty cutting up your food?	☐	☐	☐	☐	☐
16. Had difficulty holding a drink without spilling it?	☐	☐	☐	☐	☐
17. Felt depressed?	☐	☐	☐	☐	☐
18. Felt isolated and lonely?	☐	☐	☐	☐	☐
19. Felt weepy or tearful?	☐	☐	☐	☐	☐
20. Felt angry or bitter?	☐	☐	☐	☐	☐
21. Felt anxious?	☐	☐	☐	☐	☐
22. Felt worried about your future?	☐	☐	☐	☐	☐
23. Felt you had to conceal your Parkinson's from people?	☐	☐	☐	☐	☐

*Please check that you have ticked **one box for each question** before going on to the next page*

Due to having Parkinson's disease, how often during the last month have you ...

*Please tick **one box** for each question*

	Never	Occasionally	Sometimes	Often	Always or cannot do at all
24. Avoided situations which involve eating or drinking in public?	☐	☐	☐	☐	☐
25. Felt embarrassed in public due to having Parkinson's disease?	☐	☐	☐	☐	☐
26. Felt worried by other people's reaction to you?	☐	☐	☐	☐	☐
27. Had problems with your close personal relationships?	☐	☐	☐	☐	☐
28. Lacked support in the ways you need from your spouse or partner? *If you do not have a spouse or partner tick here* ☐	☐	☐	☐	☐	☐
29. Lacked support in the ways you need from your family or close friends?	☐	☐	☐	☐	☐
30. Unexpectedly fallen asleep during the day?	☐	☐	☐	☐	☐
31. Had problems with your concentration, e.g. when reading or watching TV?	☐	☐	☐	☐	☐
32. Felt your memory was bad?	☐	☐	☐	☐	☐
33. Had distressing dreams or hallucinations?	☐	☐	☐	☐	☐
34. Had difficulty with your speech?	☐	☐	☐	☐	☐

*Please check that you have ticked **one box for each question** before going on to the next page*

Due to having Parkinson's disease, how often during the last month have you ...

*Please tick **one box** for each question*

	Never	Occasionally	Sometimes	Often	Always or cannot do at all
35. Felt unable to communicate with people properly?	☐	☐	☐	☐	☐
36. Felt ignored by people?	☐	☐	☐	☐	☐
37. Had painful muscle cramps or spasms?	☐	☐	☐	☐	☐
38. Had aches and pains in your joints or body?	☐	☐	☐	☐	☐
39. Felt unpleasantly hot or cold?	☐	☐	☐	☐	☐

Please check that you have ticked one box for each question

Thank you for completing the questionnaire

The Geriatric Depression Scale

This scale is in the public domain (www.stanford.edu/~yesavage/GDS.html) and was originally developed by Dr TL Brink and Dr JA Yesavage. Choose the best answer for how you have felt over the past week:

1. Are you basically satisfied with your life? YES / **NO**
2. Have you dropped many of your activities and interests? **YES** / NO
3. Do you feel that your life is empty? **YES** / NO
4. Do you often get bored? **YES** / NO
5. Are you in good spirits most of the time? YES / **NO**
6. Are you afraid that something bad is going to happen to you? **YES** / NO
7. Do you feel happy most of the time? YES / **NO**
8. Do you often feel helpless? **YES** / NO
9. Do you prefer to stay at home, rather than going out and doing new things? **YES** / NO
10. Do you feel you have more problems with memory than most? **YES** / NO
11. Do you think it is wonderful to be alive now? YES / **NO**
12. Do you feel pretty worthless the way you are now? **YES** / NO
13. Do you feel full of energy? YES / **NO**
14. Do you feel that your situation is hopeless? **YES** / NO
15. Do you think that most people are better off than you are? **YES** / NO

Answers in bold indicate depression. Although differing sensitivities and specificities have been obtained across studies, for clinical purposes a score > 5 points is suggestive of depression and should warrant a follow-up interview. Scores > 10 are almost always depression.

APPENDIX 2
Glossary

α-synuclein – Protein forming the major component of Lewy bodies. Abnormal α-synuclein has been associated with several neurodegenerative diseases including PD.

Akathisia – Complaint of restlessness associated with fidgeting or pacing.

Akinesia – Absence of body movements.

Anosmia – Loss of the sense of smell.

Apraxia – Inability to perform a learned action despite intact comprehension, sensation and motor function.

Ballismus – Abnormal flailing movements of the limbs due to damage to the subthalamic nucleus. If unilateral this is referred to as 'hemiballismus'.

Basal ganglia – Deep brain structures concerned with cognition and control of movements, including the caudate nucleus, globus pallidus, putamen, substantia nigra and subthalamic nucleus.

Bradykinesia – Slowness of movements.

Chorea – Involuntary dance-like movements.

Cogwheeling – Rhythmic brief increase in resistance and muscle tone during passive movement about a joint.

Dopamine – A chemical produced by the brain and used to transmit impulses from one cell to another. The major neurotransmitter lost in PD.

Dyskinesia – Abnormal involuntary movements frequently seen following prolonged drug treatment for PD.

Dyspraxia – Difficulty copying gestures or performing learned actions such as dressing, despite intact comprehension and motor function.

Dystonia – Sustained muscle contraction, frequently causing twisting and repetitive movement or abnormal postures of a part of the body.

Extrapyramidal system – Refers to the basal ganglia parts of the brain concerned with *movement control*, as distinct from the 'pyramidal system', which refers to

movements under control of the corticospinal tracts.

Festination – Festination is the short shuffling gait characteristically seen in a patient with PD.

Gegenhalten – Voluntary resistance to passive movement of the limbs, typically seen in patients with frontal lobe damage.

Hemiballismus – Abnormal 'flailing' involuntary movements of the contralateral limb due to damage to the subthalamic nucleus.

Hypomimia – Decreased facial expression.

Hypophonia – Diminished voice volume.

Lewy body – Inclusions within nerve cells which are seen pathologically in PD and some related conditions.

Micrographia – Very small and scribbly handwriting commonly seen in patients with PD.

Orthostatic tremor – A rare form of tremor occurring in the legs when standing still. This is only occasionally a feature of PD.

Pyramidal system – The corticospinal and corticobulbar tracts that pass through the 'pyramidal' shaped area on the surface of the lower part of the brainstem. Lesions in this pathway produce the upper motor neuron signs of spasticity, brisk reflexes and weakness.

Seborrhoea – Increased production of sebum from the sebaceous glands of the skin.

Sialorrhoea – Drooling of saliva.

Substantia nigra – Large midbrain nucleus (part of the basal ganglia) containing dopaminergic pigmented cells, which are lost in PD.

Synkinesis – Increased muscle tone in a limb that is detected by the patient performing voluntary movements in the contralateral limb, due to overflow of muscle movements into surrounding muscle groups.

Tremor – Rhythmical, involuntary oscillatory movement of a body part.

INDEX

Numbers in **bold** *refer to figures; tables and boxes*

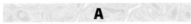

A

Ablative surgery, 116, 117, 120–121, 123, 155
  driving after, 139
Aborted embryo tissue *see* Embryonic tissue
    transplants
Activities of daily living scale, Schwab and
    England, 21, **22**
Acupuncture, 138
Addiction and L-dopa, 111
Adenosine A2A ligands, 168
Adrenal tissue transplants, 124
Adult neural stem cell transplantation, 124,
    125
Advanced PD, **20**, 21, 99–114
  assessment of patients, 111
  complications occurring, 101
  dopamine agonists, 108
  dyskinetic movements, 105
    causes, 106
    treatment, 106–108
    see also Dyskinesias
  L-dopa, 110–111
  'on/off' fluctuations, 101–105
    apomorphine, 71, 108–109, **110**
    causes, 103
    entacapone, 104–105
    freezing, 103–104
  patient questions, 113–114
  specialist clinic attendance, 112
  swallowing difficulties, 36, 111
    management, 71, 134–135
Aetiology of PD, 14–17
  environmental toxins, 16, 140, **144**, 153,
      168
  head trauma, 17
  infection, 16–17, **144**, 154
  inherited PD, 11, 13, 14–16, 19, 38, 62,
      154, 168
  patient questions, 23
Age, PD development, 13
  see also Young patients
Age Concern, 160
Ageing process and PD, 18
Agranulocytosis, 96
AIDS patients, parkinsonism, 154
Akathisia, **152**, 189
Akinesia, 27, 189

Alcohol
  essential tremor improvement, 28, 155
  patients with autonomic failure, 88
Alien hand phenomenon, **148**, 151
α_2-adrenoceptor antagonists, 168
α-adrenergic blockers, 137
α-synuclein, 4, 11, 45, 189
  in MSA, 150
  reference papers on, 166
Alzheimer's disease, 34, **43**
Amantadine, 46, 107–108, 113
  in multiple system atrophy (MSA), 150
  in progressive supranuclear palsy (PSP),
      149
Amfetamine in sleep attacks, 90
Amitriptyline, use in depression, **94**
Anatomy and physiology, 4–11
  basal ganglia, 6, **8**, 117, **118**, **119**
  dopamine, 4–6, 10–11, 189
  substantia nigra, 10–11
Animal tissue transplants, **116**, 124, 125
Ankle oedema, amantadine-induced, 108
Anosmia, 34, 189
Antibiotics, interaction with dopamine
    agonists, 73
Anticholinergic drugs
  avoiding/withdrawing in cognitive
      impairment, **91**
  side-effects
    cognitive impairment, 45, 46
    slowed bowel transit, 87
  use in
    detrusor hyperactivity, 87
    initial treatment, early PD, 69, 80
    multiple system atrophy (MSA), 150
    progressive supranuclear palsy (PSP),
        149
    reducing salivary drooling, 86
Anticonvulsants, **152**
Antidepressants
  impotence caused by, 137
  use in
    depression, 93, **94**, 95
    sleep disturbance, 89
Antiemetics, 77
  causing parkinsonism, 29, **144**, 152
  domperidone, 60, 71, 73, 76, 108, 109
  interactions with dopamine agonists, 73
Antihypertensives
  avoiding in postural hypotension, 88
  interaction with L-dopa, 78
Antiplatelet treatment in stroke, 154

E

Electromyography (EMG), external
  sphincter, 151
Embryonic tissue transplants, **116**
  neural tissue transplants, **116**, 124, **125**
  patient information, 127
  stem cell transplantation, 124, **125**
  trial with catastrophic results, 125–126
Employers, informing, 140
Encephalitis lethargica, 16–17, **144**, 154
Enemas, 87
Entacapone, 104–105
  patient information, 114
Environmental toxins
  causing parkinsonism, 16, **144**, 153
  compensation issues, 140
  patient questions, 23
  research, 168
Epidemiology
  age, PD development, 13
  causes of PD, 14–17
    see also Aetiology of PD
  gender differences, 12
  global incidence, 13–14
  prevalence of PD, 12
  reference papers on, 165
Epworth sleepiness scale, 33, **35**, 72
Equipment, adaptive, 131, 132
Erectile dysfunction, 88, 137
  patient questions, 141
Erythrocyte sedimentation rate (ESR), **61**
Erythromycin, interaction with dopamine
  agonists, 73
Essential tremor, 155
  cogwheeling, 31
  distinguishing from PD tremor, 28
  management, 80
European Parkinson's Disease Association
  web site, 159
Examination see Symptoms and problems
Executive function impairment, 46–48
  explanation for, 47–48
Exercise, 87, 134
  patient questions, 141
Extrapyramidal system, 189
Eyelid apraxia, 33
Eyes
  Kayser–Fleischer rings, iris, 60
  problems with, 33
  progressive supranuclear palsy (PSP), **147**,
    148

F

Facial expression, lack of, 27, 48, 52, 93, 189
Falls, 101
  causes, 32–33
  fractures, 135
  Parkinson-plus syndromes, **147**

preventing, 132, 133, 149
  see also Postural hypotension
Familial olivopontine-cerebellar atrophy
  (OPCA), 151
Familial progressive supranuclear palsy, 149
Family history, 16, 38
  essential tremor, 155
  see also Inherited disease
Fatigue, 71
Fava beans, 137
Favism, 137
Festination, 31–32, 189
Finger taps, bradykinesia assessment, 29
Fluctuations see 'On/off' fluctuations
Fludrocortisone in postural hypotension,
  76–77, 88, 150
Fluoro-dopa, 57–58
Fluoxetine, use in depression, **94**
Foot taps, bradykinesia assessment, 30
'Formes fruste', 3
Fractures, 135
Freezing episodes, 31, **32**, 69, 103
  apomorphine treatment, 108, 109
  causes, 103–104
  physical tricks to overcome, 133–134
  and sport, 134
Frontal cortex, 6
  and executive function impairment, 47
Funding, adaptive aids, 132

G

Gabapentin in restless legs syndrome, 89
Gadolinium, 59
Gait
  disturbances of, 27, 31–32
  improving, 132–133
Galen, 3
Gastrostomy see Percutaneous endoscopic
  gastrostomy (PEG)
GDNF see Glial derived neurotrophic factor
Gegenhalten, 31, 189
Gender and PD, 12
General practitioners (GPs), 55, 68
General reading on PD, 166
Genes
  defective, inherited PD, 11, 14–15
  essential tremor, 155
  patient questions, 23
Genetic predisposition, progressive
  supranuclear palsy, 149
Genetics, reference papers on, 165
Geriatric Depression Scale, 49, 173, 187
Geriatrician, referrals to, 55–56
Glabellar tap sign, positive, 39
Glaucoma, 33
Glial derived neurotrophic factor (GDNF),
  168

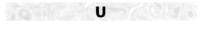

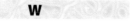